stiff quotes

Amazing class, thanks for all you have done, Nikki. Seeing a full class of 20 guys attend every week, even when Champions League football is on... wow! 'Stiff Guy' has given me a great foundation to improve my long-term wellbeing. My posture has improved dramatically and I feel stronger, more energised and more flexible every day!
Tom started 13 months ago

I have noticed better posture and balance. Yoga provides such a great balance of strength and flexibility... and Nikki's approach is a perfect balance of empathy and focus.
AV started 12 months ago

I had a very sad email this week. It was from my chiropractor, she misses me... thanks Nikki. SGY has really improved my flexibility and resilience this year.
Mike started 13 months ago

I have more flexibility and I'm also a more relaxed and have a positive attitude.
Simon started 10 months ago

My posture is stronger and more positive, a gentle ache in my muscles has replaced the pain in my back. The journey from timber to limber begins with a single stretch.
JonnyQ started two months ago

After one hour my younger. Genuine
Will started two

After only a few sessions, my long-standing lower back pain evaporated. I am more relaxed and positive in my life and it's due to this class!
Peter started two months ago

Nikki has perfected the art of engaging with all her pupils and displays endless calmness and patience!
Julian started 13 months ago

I love it! The best thing I have started for me. Thank you, Nikki.
E started two months ago

At 42 I can now touch my toes!
Chris F started four months ago

I have better stretching and posture.
CVC started one month ago

My lower back ache improved.
A started one month ago

I feel motivated to improve, as my first few sessions have left me with better breathing techniques which I can carry with me during my working day.
Andrew started this month

I feel better. It helps with my dressage too! If I miss a week, I notice the difference.
Simon started 12 months ago

I have lost one stone and become more relaxed and calm.
Mike started six months ago

My aches have disappeared and I notice a difference if I miss a week.
Steve started 14 months ago

I have better posture, increased flexibility and less back problems. And deep, deep sleeps.
Peter started 14 months ago

Fantastic way to relax and strengthen my body, which is becoming more flexible. Really enjoy it and it's a proper workout too!
DM started 11 months ago

All the little niggles and stiff back – stiffening year on year have gone! I can touch my toes and continue to feel improvements each time. Take it at your own speed, weekly work and just feel yourself get younger! Enjoy.
Michael started 11 months ago

I feel more flexible, less old, and I now have some moves I can use for those days when I'm all seized up.
Dan started 14 months ago

I feel stronger, fitter and more 'together' (and my back works)!
Harry started four months ago

I feel more flexible and relaxed after each class and have felt the improvement and benefit over the year since I started.
Chris started 14 months ago

Great for reducing stress and feel like it's added years to my life.
Mike started 12 months ago

Amazing class and teacher. First time at yoga and I'm totally hooked.
Simon started 12 months ago

I have improved balance and concentration. I am learning new moves and it's enjoyable. I feel progress and I'm loosening up slowly.
Paul started three months ago

Bob's thoughts on this book: "I'll be honest with you, I thought it was superb. I found it exhilarating and a very interesting read."
Bob started two months ago

Neil's thoughts on the book: "Really good and a welcome addition to the beginner's yoga market."
Neil started eight months ago

Mike's thoughts on the book: "Absolutely love it. Well-written and informative, I expect to see it on the bestseller list."
Mike started six months ago

REGAIN YOUR TWENTYSOMETHING SELF IN 30 DAYS

stiff guy yoga

NIKKI LYNDS-XAVIER

Matador
9 Priory Business Park,
Wistow Road, Kibworth Beauchamp,
Leicestershire. LE8 0RX
Tel: 0116 279 2299
Email: books@troubador.co.uk
Web: www.troubador.co.uk/matador
Twitter: @matadorbooks

ISBN 978 1838590 666

British Library Cataloguing in Publication Data.
A catalogue record for this book is available from the British Library.

Printed and bound by CPI Group (UK) Ltd, Croydon, CR0 4YY
Typeset in 11pt Benton Sans by Troubador Publishing Ltd, Leicester, UK

Matador is an imprint of Troubador Publishing Ltd

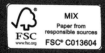

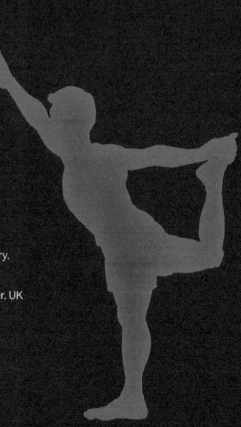

much love...

My husband Bill for his constant support, encouragement and wisdom during my lawyer-to-yogi morphosis... and my continuing journey.

My good friend Jeff Taylor, founder of *Courier Magazine*, for the idea to write this book and then encouraging me to do so.

Stiff Guys – Peter North, Tom Monaghan, Mike Humphries, Mike Wooles, Bob Dalton and Neil Morgan, whose enthusiasm and thoughts on this book spurred me onward.

Yoga virgins – Gary Winslade, Ian Chambers, Gill Rashpal, Andrew McMillan, Nik Henshaw, and Nicolas Michel for trialling the 30 Day Build and providing me with invaluable feedback.

Kevin, Helen, Sally and Matt of New Energy Yoga in Winchester for trusting in me and allowing me to grow the Stiff brand at their beautiful yoga studio.

Tracey Rich, Ganga White and Sven Holcomb of the White Lotus Foundation in Santa Barbara who honed my yoga and teaching skills, gently breaking through my English reserve to give me the confidence to be a yogi. And for their continued support and friendship despite their hectic schedules.

Karen Percival of Birch Tree Yoga for teaching and inspiring me in those early years.

And finally, to the Stiffs who bravely stepped through the studio door to give Stiff Guy Yoga a go, returning week on week. It still gives me a warm feeling looking around the class and seeing so many faces from original Team Stiff. I am beyond proud of you. Thank you for all your hard work in class, and your contribution to the quotes within these pages. Without you, this book would never have been written.

namaste

contents

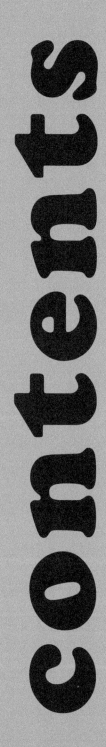

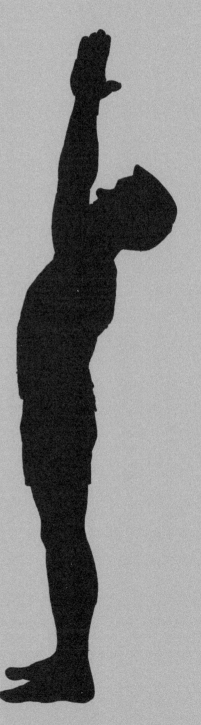

Suddenly, men everywhere are doing it – elite sportsmen, celebrities, work colleagues and friends. Large corporations now offer it as part of their health care and even construction workers after a hard day's work are heading to yoga studios. What the hell is going on?!

Men have cottoned on to the fact that strength without flexibility is a weakness. Even Her Majesty's Army have embraced yoga (more about that later). And it's not just middle-aged men who are struggling. Young men who have built muscle in the gym or whilst doing sport are finding that their mobility has significantly decreased, and have turned to yoga to unlock their body's potential.

The world of yoga is confusing, though. So many different types. Classes online or in a studio or gym. And social media is awash with teachers in seemingly impossible positions, perched precariously in front of a sunset or bowl of fruit. It's really off-putting, and it's often misleading. And it's

why I've written this guide to yoga for men. For you. That's why you'll only occasionally see pictures of me on social media because it's not about me; it's about you, it's about Stiff Guy Yoga (SGY).

This book is written with the total beginner in mind, but also for the guy who feels he's never really fully understood the mechanics and needs some further guidance.

Look, here's my pitch. Take on the 30 Day Build, and in return you will regain your twentysomething self.

This sounds like a huge promise, but I've seen the results time and time again. And the feedback has not just been from happy students, but also their delighted partners who have hugged me in the street. You'll see some of the quotes from my rejuvenated students within these covers.

So what does it mean to have your twentysomething self back? Well first of all there's your weight. And then there's your posture. And your flexibility, of course. And your zeal for life... you get the picture.

The anecdotal weight loss of my overweight students, attending one class a week for nine months without dieting is 0.5 – 1 stone. Obviously, achieving your twentysomething body within 30 days is going to depend on your starting point, but it can be done. However, regardless of weight loss, you will regain your youthful zip. Your posture will dramatically improve, your stamina will increase, your blood pressure should be in its healthy range and your zeal for life will return. In short, you will feel like YOU again. What is more, in 30 days you'll establish an enjoyable habit that will

extend your health span for years to come.

The great thing about yoga is almost anyone can do it. It doesn't require you to set record distances or destroy yourself into a sweaty heap in a group spin session. But of course, like any exercise program, I can't know what your current health is like. Before you start any exercise program or make a big change in your health, you should check with your doctor beforehand. This is especially important if you have any existing medical conditions or a concern about your health. And if you have injuries, getting your physiotherapist involved early is always a good idea too.

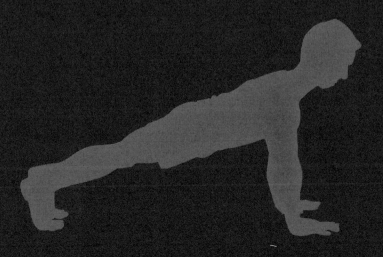

how it all began

"What do you mean you can't put your socks on without sitting down?!" I asked a bunch of my male friends. "Why? When did this happen?"

And so the seed for Stiff Guy Yoga was planted, with the first class on 5 January 2018. I expected only a few blokes to turn up, as it's scary attending your first yoga class, right? Am I joining a cult, a religion, hippiedom or worse... do I have to give up meat? But in they came, and within weeks there was a waiting list. The results were talking.

Class maxed out at 26 mats, and with longer limbs to accommodate, teaching required mindful supervision of these yoga virgins. The guys had total focus, giving it 100% and within six weeks, the first student touched his toes. On average, every fortnight another reached the floor, some for the first time in 30 years. The joy that brought to us both was palpable. Their partners stopping me in the street, thanking me for the change it had made to their loved ones' wellbeing.

The guys were now hooked on yoga, keen to progress and learn more. As well as gaining flexibility, strength and tone, many were losing significant amounts of weight. Shoulders were back, heads were high and their eyes were bright. They looked well, and I noticed they were looking younger. They were regaining their youthful bounce.

Don't get me wrong, it wasn't all about toes. Each week we focused on a different part of the body; the problem areas for Stiff Guys – backs, hamstrings, hips, core and shoulders. Mixing things up to keep it interesting. My intention was that classes should be physical but thoughtful, challenging and fun. And that they would sweat, banishing the notion that yoga was housewives' choice.

When I started SGY, the regular studio classes had a few men in, but many had none. I was determined this would change. The studio's owners admired the ambition, said it would never happen but provided their full support, for which I am eternally grateful. By the summer of 2018, my mixed classes had reached almost fifty-fifty, including the hot yoga class. Mission accomplished. Thank you gentlemen.

As a direct result of the Stiffs (yes, there's a name for you) spreading the word and not wanting to be left out, the ladies demanded Stiff Girl (but that's another story).

the girl in the class

I got into yoga in 2007. I was three stone overweight and a partner in a law firm. So long hours and food on the go. I was good at diets though, I like a goal; but the minute I hit my target weight, the weight crept back on. I knew I had to change my lifestyle if I was to get out of this annual dieting cycle. I happened to read an article by a New York photographer who was renowned for taking nude portraits. To put her subjects at ease, she would chat to them about their hobbies, and she realised that those with enviable bodies all had one thing in common – they did yoga. That was reason enough for me to try it.

Back then it was hard to find a good class outside of London. So there were numerous occasions when I wanted to bolt for the door of the village hall or sports centre I found myself in. (I was actually asked to leave one because I had a fit of giggles.) After a bit of research, I purchased a DVD and taught myself the basics at home over a few weeks; and I quickly became hooked. If you're interested in exactly who and what led me here, visit www.stiffguyyoga.co.uk and download my links list. You can even purchase some of this stuff directly from my site.

The weight gradually and naturally started to drop off. I also noticed that I was making different food choices; my body seemed to want more natural food. I've been a fish-eating veggie since my teens. I was a squeamish child and, to the horror of my medical family, I stopped eating meat. It was rare to find veggie options back then, so I swallowed a lot of processed carbs and that undoubtedly led to the weight gain. Yoga seemed to flick a subconscious switch and the idea of processed food no longer appealed. I also noticed that I was drinking less alcohol; again a subconscious decision. It sounds

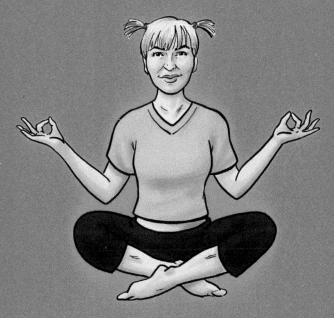

ridiculous, I know (I get that), but my students have the same experience.

For the next decade, I practised yoga two to three days a week, both at home and in classes in the UK and abroad. I started selecting holidays based on their yoga offering, and I covered a lot of countries and styles of yoga on that basis. I then reached a point where I wanted to advance my practise further and teacher training was an option suggested to me by my teacher, even though I had no plans to teach. So I sat down one afternoon in a local café with my laptop and I started researching yoga schools. As the rain lashed against the window, I trawled through all the top schools in Asia, Europe and Australia, but none of them offered exactly what I was looking for. I was just shutting my laptop when an email pinged through and I opened it. It was from the White Lotus Foundation (WLF) asking me if I'd considered teacher training. I couldn't believe it. I'd not got as far as searching American and Canadian schools, as I'd run out of time and in any event, the WLF don't use algorithms looking for search patterns. They rarely advertise, as they don't need to. I remembered years before signing up for newsletters, but I'd received them only very occasionally. More than a little spooked, I rushed off to a yoga class I'd booked, deciding to reflect on this development on the mat.

There was a new receptionist on the desk and as she spoke, I felt the blood drain out of my face. She was American. She asked me if I was OK, so I hastily explained the coincidence and as I was finishing this voice behind me shouted, "Just book it!" I turned around to see a friend that I'd never bumped into before at the studio, and who I'd heard was planning to train to be a yoga teacher. Decision made, straight after class I headed home, completed the WLF application forms and sent them off. I didn't for one moment think I'd be accepted, as the WLF is one of the best, if not the best yoga school in America. The list of renowned yoga teachers and students that they have worked with is mind-blowing. So to find myself on day one of the WLF training course sitting with the other students who had come from all over America, was surreal. At the end of the first day, as I dragged my aching body into bed, I did wonder if I'd made a terrible mistake. Despite having increased my daily practise, I wasn't sure I was strong enough to complete day two, let alone the weeks that lay ahead.

Long story short, I got stronger day by day, made lifelong friends with both the students and the teachers, and loved every minute of my time there. I passed all my exams and, despite a drawer full of academic qualifications back home, my yoga teaching certificate is the one I am most proud of.

Returning home was a shock, as I'd been away for a few months. Grappling with the dramatic drop in temperature, driving on the left and feeling weird wearing socks again, I stumbled into the yoga studio, where I bumped into Helen, one of the directors. Still jet-lagged, I found myself agreeing to audition to be one of their teachers, and before the week was out, I'd passed and was booked onto the timetable. I'd agreed on condition that I could teach a men's only class, which everyone was pleased about until I announced the name... Stiff Guy Yoga. I was adamant I wasn't changing the name, but not everyone liked it. So the team took a vote and I won by just one vote. And the rest, as they say, is history.

Now fast forward and it's not just office-bound guys I teach. I've worked with everyone from the British Armed Forces to the Emergency Services around the country. I was hugely impressed with Commanding Officer Nick MacKenzie's foresight as to the advantage yoga might bring to the soldiers, having

never tried it himself. And it is to both the soldiers and their officers' credit that they embraced the challenge, working hard to combine flexibility with their existing strength and endurance.

You know, like a lot of 'fit' men, cardiovascular health and strength doesn't necessarily translate to flexibility. These guys were some of the stiffest I've ever met! So I figure if what we're doing works for these elite guys, imagine what it can do for you too.

My yoga journey continues at a pace, and I am so very grateful to find myself on this path, and to feel like I am making a difference. It's an unusual feeling, as a lawyer, making people happy!

some stiff stories

The names have been changed to protect the innocent.

Jon – over the years the weight had crept on and, with little time outside of business and family commitments, Jon hadn't exercised regularly since his twenties, except for the annual skiing holiday and last minute prep. Jon's friend was a yoga teacher and she had been on at him for years to give it a go, but she wasn't local. So when he heard of the Stiff Guy class, he thought now's the time to try it.

Taking a mat at the back of the class, Jon joined the other Stiffs six months ago. He found the first class tough – everyone does – but he really enjoyed the vibe and slept surprisingly soundly that night. And he has returned every week since, save for holidays. Today he is a stone lighter without dieting, he looks considerably younger, to the extent that everyone's commenting, and reports that he feels so much more relaxed.

Jack – joined the Stiffs two months ago, informing me that he'd suffered with lower back pain for years and he'd tried everything. I hear this a lot; maybe as many as one in three Stiffs report historic back pain, injury or even surgery. And all are still suffering a form of discomfort or pain, with some having to take time off work.

I advised Jack to work to his edge. Discomfort is okay but pain isn't – it's feedback telling you to stop. So take it gently, and with time, the muscles supporting the spine will strengthen and flexibility will return.

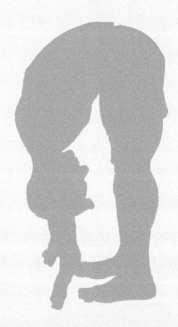

After the first class, Jack said that he felt some sensitivity in his back. It felt like it had been exercised but it wasn't painful, though he was reserving judgement until the following morning when he would know for sure.

The following week, Jack was back on the mat and reported that he'd slept really well and been fine in the morning, with just awareness that his back had had a workout. And so, Jack became a regular in the Stiff class. Eight weeks on, Jack caught me at the end of class to say that he no longer has any back pain, utterly delighted after all these years to have finally found a cure in yoga.

And this is not an isolated case. I've lost count of the number of students who are now pain free.

And I'll quickly tell you about one of my Stiff Girls who joined the women's class. She was on the waiting list for a new hip... I say was, because 12 months of weekly Stiff Girl Yoga and her astonished doctor confirmed she no longer needs one! She was thrilled and so was I. Amazing.

I digress. So back to the guys.

Adam – is six foot and then some, but when I met him his shoulders were hunched forward. He commutes daily and is seated for much of the day. He came along to one of my beginner's workshops, where I run through all the basics (for workshop details go to www.stiffguyyoga.co.uk). He was very conscious of his lack of flexibility and, having tried the workshop, thought Stiff Guy was worth a shot, and booked a block of 15 classes.

The first class confirmed to Adam that he did need to improve his flexibility, but also his balance, as he struggled with the balance poses. A few weeks in and I noticed Adam walk into reception with his shoulders back and his head held high. I asked him if I was imagining it and he said no. He'd also noticed he was more upright. Then at six weeks, at the end of class, Adam told me he'd just touched his toes for the first time in 30 years. We both stood there grinning at each other. It was a moment I will never forget.

And today, he's in class two to three times a week and he's nailing those balances.

Last, but by no means least Tim – one of my original Stiffs who attended my first class because his wife had bought him 10 Stiff Guy classes for Christmas. (Actually, quite a few of the original Stiffs joined because their partners signed them up, and they're still in class.) Tim told me he was sceptical that it would make a difference and being knackered after work, he would rather have a glass of wine, but said he'd give Stiff Guy a few weeks. And to his credit, he didn't do it half-heartedly, he gave it his all.

Tim continued to come to class once a week and in week 10 he told me he'd just booked a block of 15 classes. He quietly admitted to me that when I'd first met him he felt constantly tired and he'd resigned himself to the fact that he was ageing, and it was all downhill from now on (mid-forties). But to his amazement, Stiff Guy had given him his energy back. He'd even agreed to do a cycling weekend with a group of friends and, having just bought a bike, could I give him some post-training poses to do at home?

Then in the summer, I was walking down the high street with my earphones in, when this woman ran in front of me. She was talking and pointing to a man queuing at a stall who was waving at me. It was Tim. With my earphones now

out, I could hear her thanking me for rejuvenating her husband. She'd been so worried about him; she was convinced he was depressed but he wouldn't talk about it. In desperation, she'd bought the yoga classes and had fully anticipated him refusing to go, but the name of the class had made him laugh out loud.

And the rest is history.

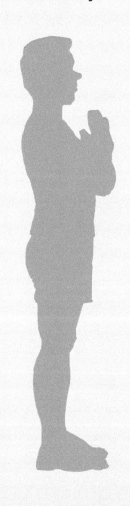

These illustrated poses are annotated with some top tips, but for more in-depth guidance you can watch my videos at www.stiffguyyoga.co.uk, where I take you through the poses step-by-step.

the poses guide

backbend

- Inhaling, take your hands to prayer overhead, and lengthen
- Keeping your legs straight, push your pelvis forward and reach your hands back
- Look up at your hands, if your neck allows

bridge

- With your knees and feet hip-width apart, plant your feet close to your sit bones
- Engage your core and lift your hips
- Squeeze your thighs up and together
- Keep weight in your heels and shoulders

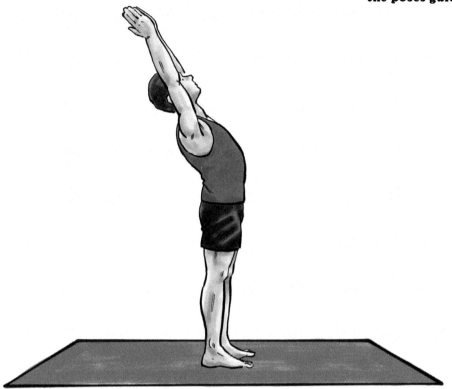

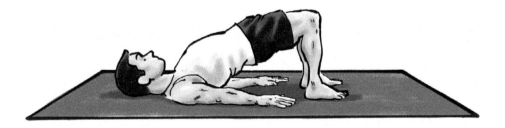

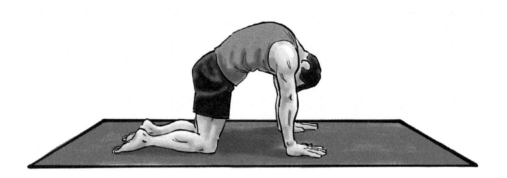

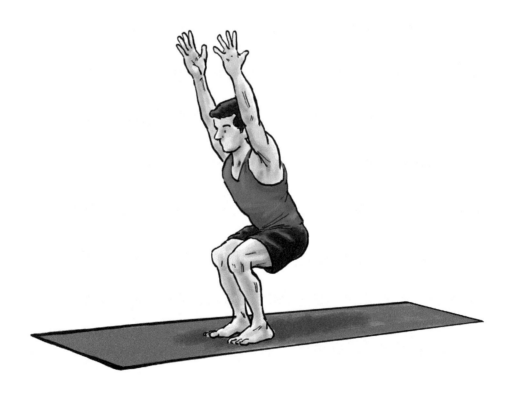

cat

- Exhaling, tuck your naval to your spine and your chin to your chest
- Arch into your shoulders, pushing into your hands
- Round your back

chair

- Place your feet hip-width apart, with your weight in your heels
- Lengthen your arms upwards, palms facing each other and sink down
- Don't tip forwards – it's as if you are sitting in a chair
- Squeeze your thighs together

child's

- Hands are shoulder-width apart and fingers splayed
- Reach into your hands and push your shoulder blades back and down
- Weight is towards your sit bones
- Keep alignment from your fingers all the way down your spine

cobra

- Keep your feet together and your bent elbows in by your sides
- Press your feet into the mat, applying gentle pressure into your hands
- Engage your core and lengthen your spine
- Squeeze your shoulder blades back and down

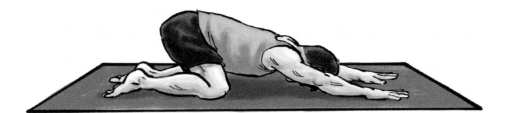

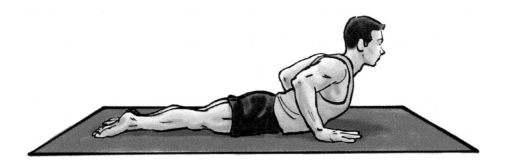

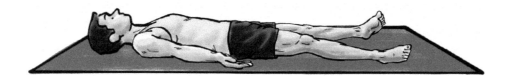

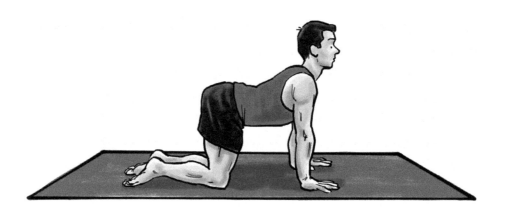

corpse

- Take your feet as wide as your mat, with your heels in, your toes drop outwards
- Hands' palms up by your sides
- Shoulder blades are back and down
- Chin very slightly tucked
- Relax

cow

- Inhaling, let your stomach sag
- Expand your chest and arch your sit bones back
- Look up

dancer

- Engage your core and grab the inside of your foot
- Tilt, keeping your hips facing forwards and your standing leg straight
- Kick your foot into your hand
- Reach upwards with your front hand to counterbalance
- Repeat on the other side

dancer prep

- Engage your core, reach back and grab the inside of your foot
- Keep your hips facing forwards and your standing leg straight
- Reach upwards with your other hand and lengthen
- Repeat on the other side

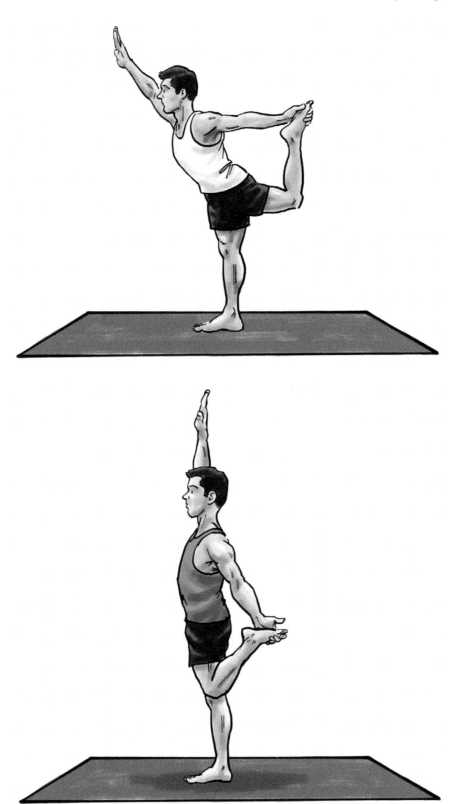

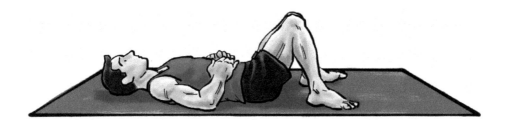

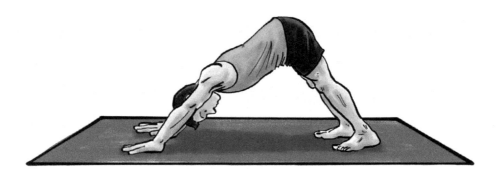

deep lower back release

- Take your feet as wide as your mat and drop your knees together
- Feel your lower back gently arch
- Place your hands on your stomach
- Inhale deeply. Exhale to empty and feel your pelvis tilt towards you and your lower back sink into the mat. Repeat three times

down dog

- Place your feet hip-width apart, with weight in your heels
- Draw your shoulder blades down and together to open your chest
- Draw your stomach towards your thighs
- With your ears beside your biceps, relax your neck and look at your feet

forward and backward spinal rocking

- If you can, cross your ankles and take hold of your feet or ankles, that is the more advanced option
- If you struggle to reach your feet, keep your shins, ankles and feet side by side and hold your shins instead
- Rock yourself forward and backward to massage your spine

forward fold

- Keep your feet planted hip-width apart
- Hinge forward at your hips, with your chest drawing towards your thighs
- To release any lower back tension, soften your knees or bend your knees
- Relax your neck, so there is no strain

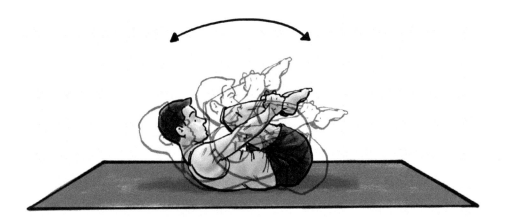

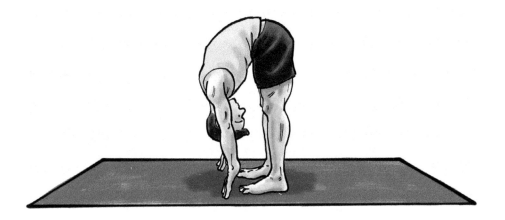

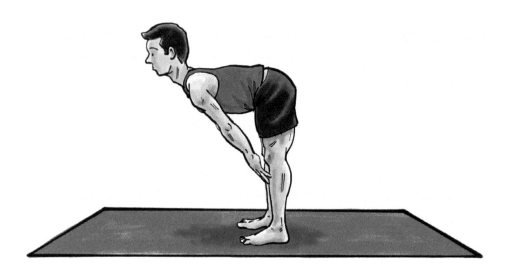

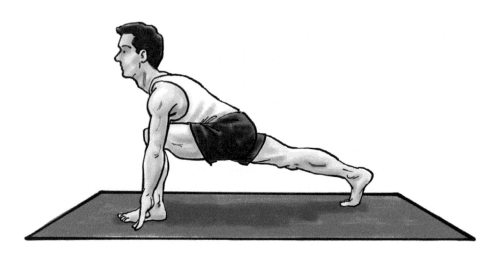

half fold

- With straight arms, push into your hands on your knees or shins
- Maintain a flat back
- Expand your chest and look forward

high lunge

- Keep your front knee directly above your ankle
- Lift and expand your chest
- Keep your back leg straight and push into the heel
- Engage your core
- Repeat on the other side

locust

- Go gently as this is a strong pose. Maybe just lift the upper body. And then lift just the legs, keeping the upper body on the mat
- Engage your core and expand your chest
- Squeeze your shoulder blades back and down
- Lift your arms and legs as high as you can, whilst lengthening
- Lift your chin and breathe

low lunge

- Keep your front knee above your ankle
- Square your hips and expand your chest
- With your weight in your front foot, look forward
- Repeat on the other side

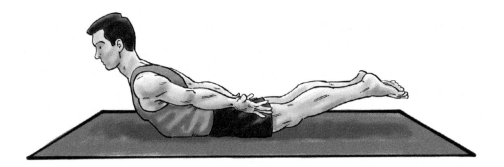

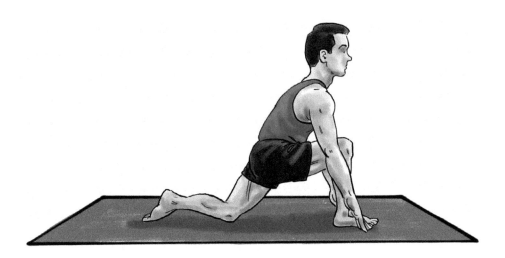

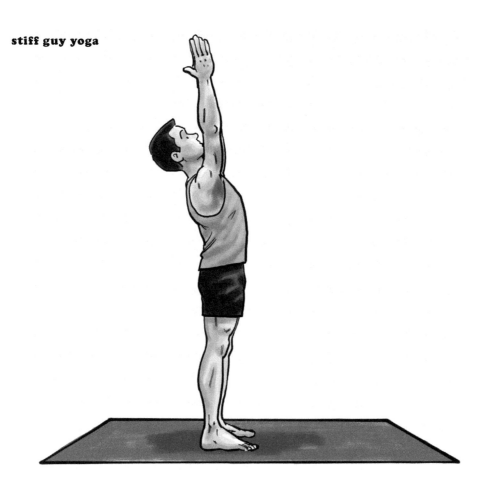

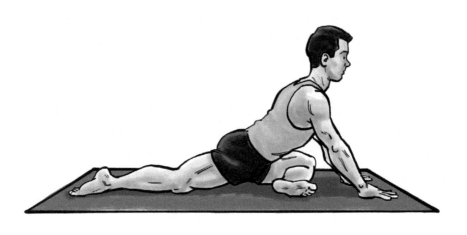

mountain

- Keep your feet planted hip-width apart
- Ensure your hips are square forward
- Inhaling, lift your arms overhead to prayer hands, draw your rib cage away from your hips

pigeon

- Keep your hips square forward and your back leg straight
- Laterally rotate your front knee to the side but only as far as is comfortable
- Exhaling, relax down over the front leg, softening your hips to the floor. You can rest your forehead on stacked clasped hands or stacked forearms
- Repeat on the other side

plank

- Place your hands under your shoulders, with your middle fingers pointing forward
- Squeeze your shoulder blades back and down, and expand your chest
- Ensure weight is across the whole of your hand, whilst extending back into your heels

pose of eight curves

- From plank, drop both your knees to the mat, then place your chest and chin between your hands. Sit bones stay in the air
- Slide your chest through your hands, so your pelvis comes to the mat
- Untuck toes and keep your elbows in by your sides

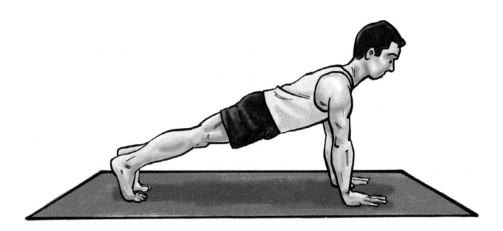

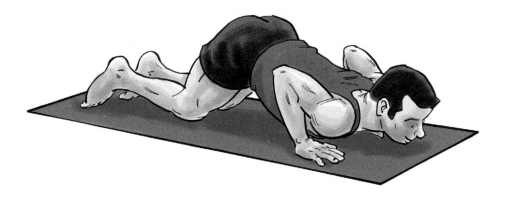

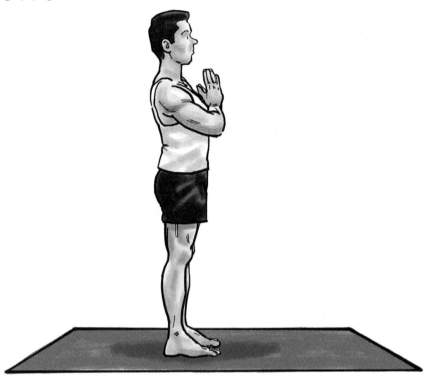

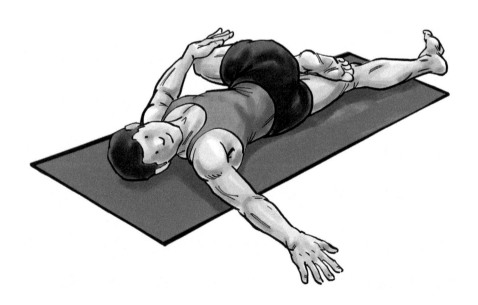

prayer

- Exhale and bring your hands to heart centre
- Draw your shoulder blades back and down
- Ensure your hips are square forward

reclined single leg twist

- Keep your shoulders on the mat
- Look out over your outstretched hand
- Feel a gentle lower back release
- Repeat on the other side

reclined stretch

- Keep your toes pointed, and your hands reaching to lengthen
- Take your right hand and right foot an inch or two off the mat and stretch. Repeat on the left, and then repeat on the diagonals
- (This book is obviously designed for men but just in case a woman is doing this pose – do not do the diagonal stretch if there is any chance you may be pregnant.)

seated cross-leg twist

- Inhaling, press into the hand by the base of your spine and lengthen upwards
- Exhaling, use the hand on your knee to rotate your chest in the opposite direction, and look over the shoulder
- Inhale and exhale three times on each side
- Change front leg and repeat to the other side

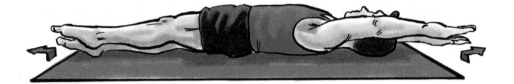

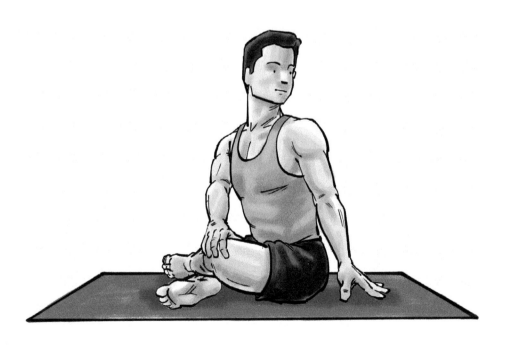

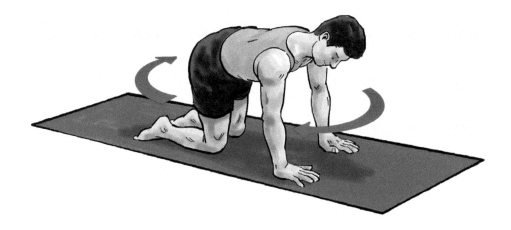

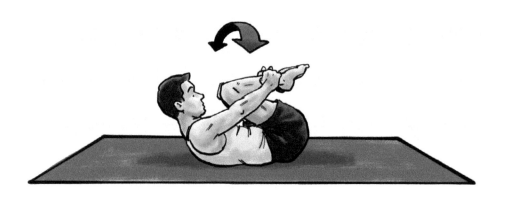

sexy kitty

- Take your right hip back to right heel, then shift your weight so your left hip comes over your left heel. Lean forwards over your left hand and then shift your weight over to your right hand
- Complete three clockwise circles and then complete three anticlockwise

sideways spinal rocking

- Keep shins, ankles and feet side by side and hold your shins or knees
- Gently rock left to right, massaging your spine

single knee hug

- Inhale, bring your knee into your chest and hug, with your feet flexed
- Keep your shoulders back and down, and your head on the mat
- Engage your core and breathe deeply
- Repeat on the other side

sphinx

- Forearms are shoulder-width apart and elbows under your shoulders
- Press into your forearms and tops of your toes
- Squeeze your shoulder blades back and down
- Extend your chest bone and head upwards

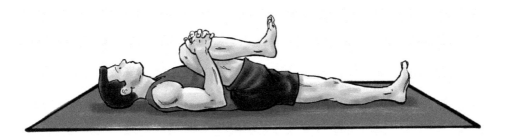

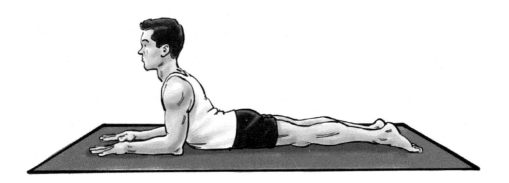

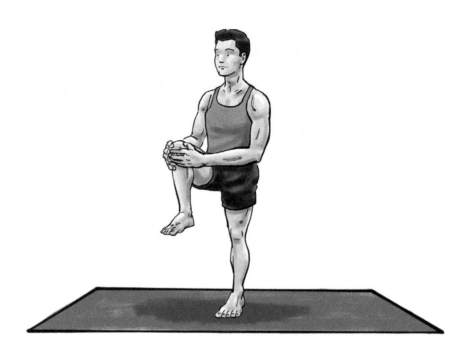

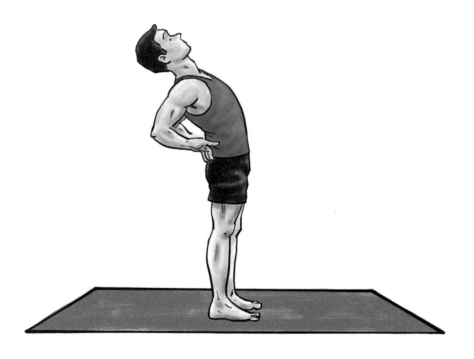

standing knee balance

- Straighten your standing leg and hug your other knee into your chest
- Draw your shoulder blades back and down
- Engage your core
- Repeat on the other side

supported back bend

- Keep your feet planted hip-width apart
- Little fingers are either side of the base of your spine
- Squeeze your elbows and shoulder blades together
- Gently push your pelvis forward and look up and back, if your neck allows

table top

- Knees and feet are hip-width apart
- Hands are directly under shoulders, fingers splayed and middle finger pointing forward
- Keep your back flat

tree

- Straighten your standing leg and engage your core
- Keep your hips square forward but tighten the glute of the bent leg to draw the knee out to the side
- Press your foot into your thigh, shin or ankle
- Repeat on the other side

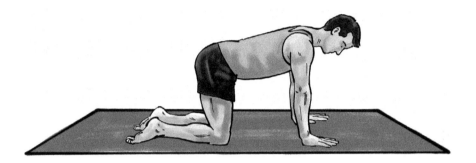

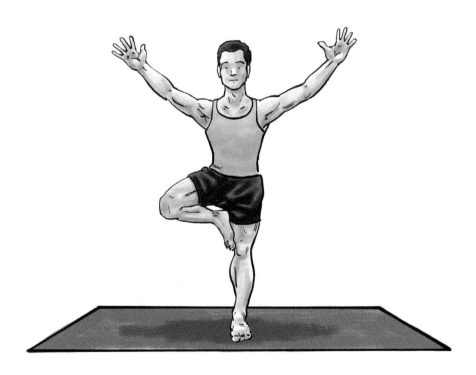

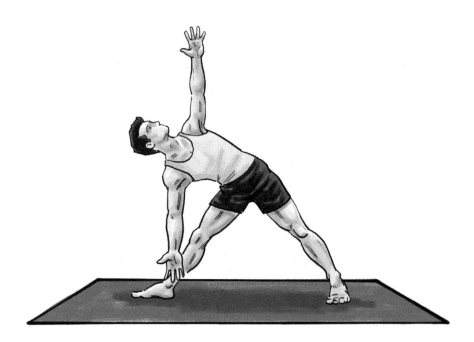

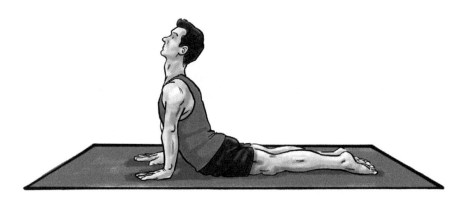

triangle

- Place your feet in a 'T' formation, with the heel of your front foot in line with the centre of the arch of your back foot
- Expand your chest. Reach and look upwards if your neck allows
- Engage your core
- Do not lean on the front leg
- Repeat on the other side

up dog

- Place your hands under your shoulders, and straighten your arms
- Lengthen your chest bone upwards
- Squeeze your shoulder blades together and expand your chest
- Press the tops of your feet into the mat

warrior i

- Feet are two thirds of a stride apart, approximately hip-width. The back foot is at a 45° angle pressing into the outside edge of your foot
- Front knee is bent and directly above your ankle
- Hips are square forward
- Lengthen arms and sink in to your hips, keeping your weight centred
- Repeat on the other side

warrior ii

- Place your feet in a 'T' formation, with the heel of your front foot in line with the centre of the arch of your back foot
- Ensure your front knee is directly above your ankle and your back leg is straight
- Squeeze your shoulder blades back and down
- Look out over your front middle finger
- Repeat on the other side

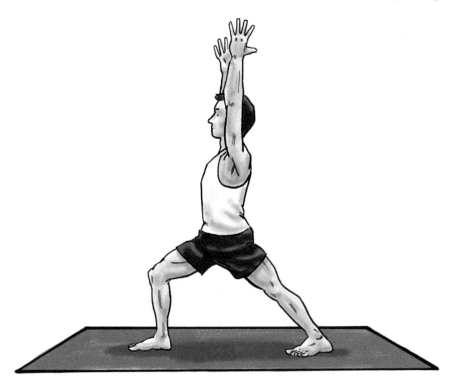

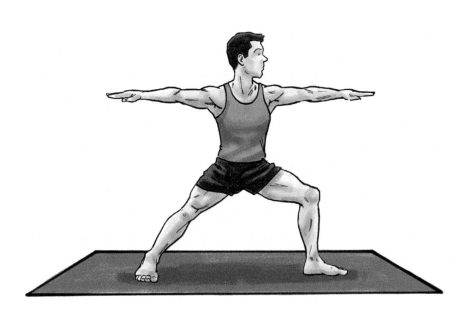

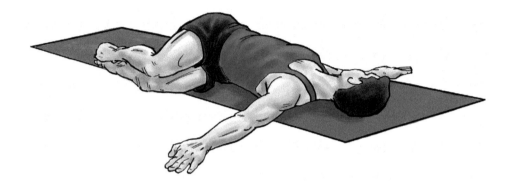

windscreen wiper twist

- With your feet and knees hip-width apart, roll in the same direction onto the edges of your feet and drop your knees towards the floor
- Look in the opposite direction to your knees and relax
- Feel a gentle back release
- Repeat on the other side

I have designed six routines of approximately 10 to 60 minutes which, for simplicity, I've labelled Red, Pink, Blue, Green, Orange and Yellow. Red being the shortest and Yellow the longest (see the table on page 46). Each of the 30 days is assigned a colour and on pages 48–89, the routines are outlined and illustrated for ease of reference when practising. However, you may prefer to follow a video, so I have prepared six videos with their corresponding colour labels to aid your 30 Day Build. You can access these via www.stiffguyyoga.co.uk.

Yoga at its simplest is breath and spine. Yes, there is considerably more to it, and always more to learn, which is one of the reasons why I love it. This book is designed for the total beginner, so let's keep things simple. We won't be using the traditional Sanskrit names for the poses. I will instead be focusing on teaching you the essential poses and breath work.

I do not believe that pain should form any part of your yoga experience. If you feel pain, it's feedback telling you to ease off. It is important that you learn to listen to your body. I recommend that you aim for 75% of your edge and then work towards 100%. By edge, I mean the edge of your comfort zone in a pose.

So it's going to vary from pose to pose, and it will be different on each side of your body, and from day to day. You'll notice the time of day will also make a difference, as we are generally tighter in the morning and looser at the end of the day.

The great thing about yoga is that you are working to your edge and not someone else's goal. Leave your ego at the door. It is small, incremental progress through practise that in time manifests itself in previously inconceivable results.

Yoga builds awareness of your body, its limitations and its potential. So do not beat yourself up because other guys can do something and you can't. It will probably happen, but it takes time to open gently and safely. Instead start to take note of where you are in your body each day and honour it. Work with it, rather than fight against it. You may never get into some positions like the Lotus position (and many yogis can't) because anatomically it's impossible for you. I can't do the splits. I can get close but then it's bone on bone and pushing further is just wearing away my joints, so I don't. There are literally thousands of poses, so not being able to master some is no biggy.

30
days

day 1 – prep

Purchase a yoga mat

You are going to need a yoga mat. They are the only essential piece of yoga equipment that you need, but don't be tempted to buy an expensive one at this stage, as it's not necessary. Prices can vary enormously and some of the very cheap ones look good but be sure to check the grip or you'll be sliding all over the place when you warm up. The mat needs to provide you with some cushioning but not too much – you're not sleeping on it. And your hands need to stick to the mat and not slide when they are sweaty.

There are plenty of reputable yoga mat retailers out there; be guided by user reviews if you are buying online and can't actually try the mat. Alternatively, if you'd like a Stiff Guy mat, go to www.stiffguyyoga.co.uk.

The other thing you'll need is some comfortable clothing that you can bend in and don't mind getting sweaty. So track pants or shorts, and a tee or vest. And no socks – which always comes as a shock to British guys who have to be coaxed out of their socks at their first class. You need your bare feet gripping the mat. We're going to stimulate all those nerves in your feet and restore your balance and agility. Trust me, you could injure yourself with socks on. I'm not a fan of yoga socks, as they are still no substitute for the soles of your feet.

Learn the breathing technique

This is really important.

There are a few different types of yogic breathing which are all valuable tools. But to start you on your yoga journey, I'm going to take a straightforward approach and have you concentrate on improving the depth and speed of your breath.

Breath practise is important because it will improve your control and lung capacity, which will increase your available oxygen, strengthen your yoga and release stress. Filling the body with oxygen raises the alkalinity of the body and so combats inflammation in all tissue, helping you to move comfortably without pain.

To start with, lie down on your back and place your hands on your stomach. Inhale deeply through your nose and feel your diaphragm move down and your stomach rise and then fall as you breathe out. Think of Buddha's big round belly. Next, repeat, but once your stomach has inflated, see if you can keep inhaling to fill your chest and your lungs before exhaling. Try this again, and see if you can take in even more breath and feel your collarbone rise after your lungs fill before exhaling. Take your time over inhaling and exhaling. No rush.

It is important to practise your breathing at the start of your daily yoga practise and then try and incorporate it into your yoga. It will make a big difference to your yoga, providing a meditative rhythm and focus, allowing you to go deeper into poses and hold them for longer. Once you've mastered it lying down, you can try it seated or standing. And as you improve, increase the inhale from two to three seconds to five seconds or more.

It is something I found very difficult to start with, but I persisted until I had a eureka moment when my breathing and movement harmonised together, and it changed my yoga forever. My students also struggle to keep it going throughout their practise but when they noticed they've stopped the technique, they just pick it up again. And that is what you must aim for. Rome wasn't built in a day.

1	2	3	4	5	6	7
8	9	10	11	12	13	14
15	16	17	18	19	20	21
22	23	24	25	26	27	28
29	30					

the six routines

For help with the rhythm, number of reps and length of time to hold poses, go to my website www.stiffguyyoga.co.uk for guided videos. If you don't have access to the internet, then aim to hold poses for three to five breaths and move at a pace comfortable for you. And importantly, always repeat the sun salutations on both the left and right sides, i.e. first lead with the right leg, then repeat the salutation leading with the left leg.

And remember, some of these poses are stronger than others, so go slowly and listen to your body.

the
build

red

Reclined Stretch – Sideways Spinal Rocking – Single Knee Hug – Forward and Backward Spinal Rocking – Seated Cross-leg Twist – Child's – Table Top – Cow – Cat – Sexy Kitty – Child's

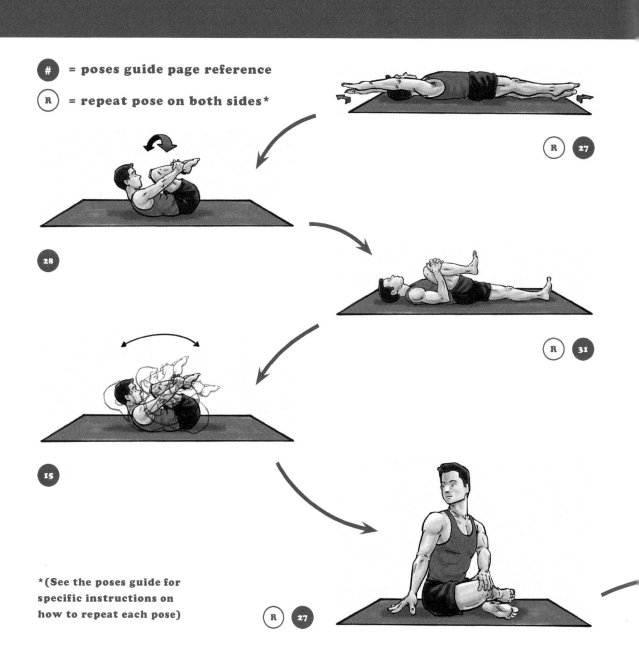

= poses guide page reference

R = repeat pose on both sides*

R 27

28

R 31

15

*(See the poses guide for specific instructions on how to repeat each pose)

R 27

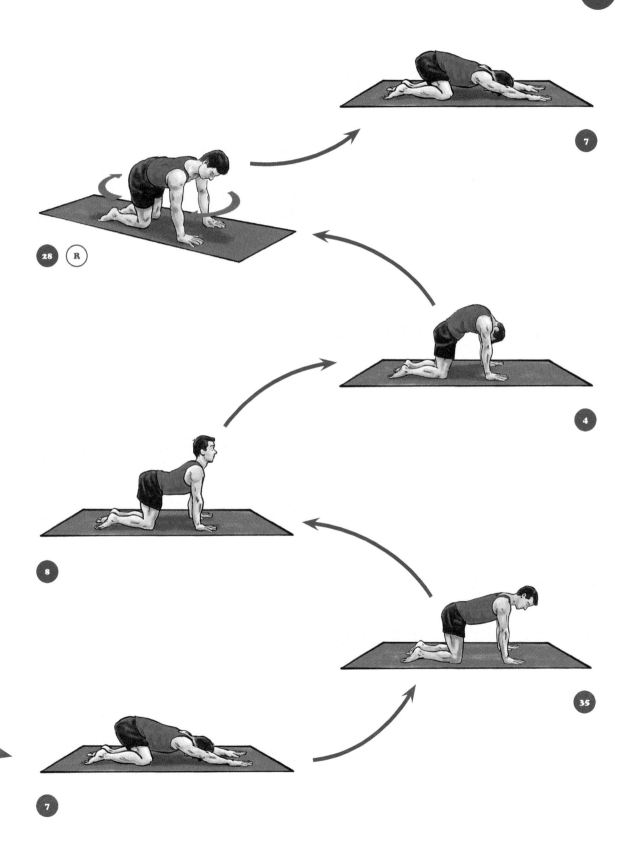

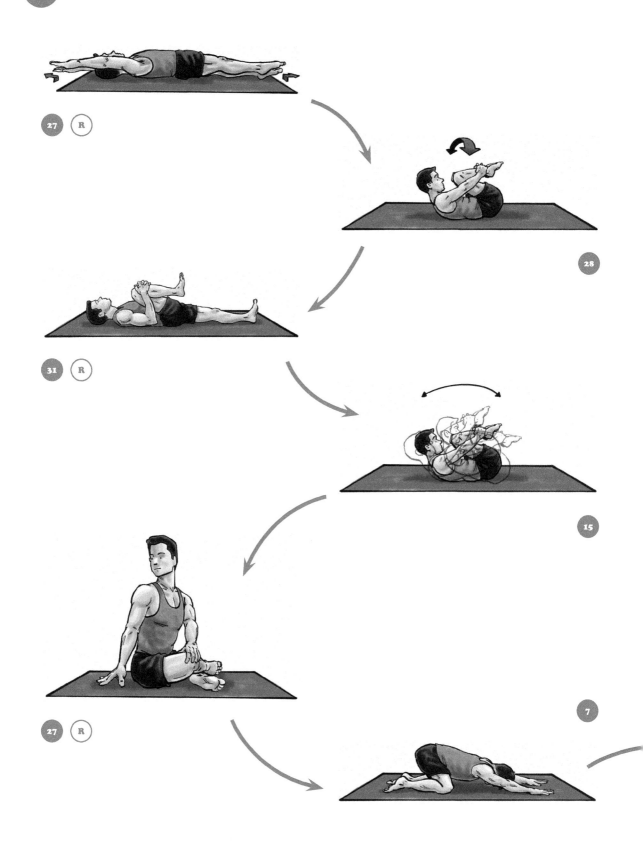

27 R

28

31 R

15

27 R

7

pink

Reclined Stretch – Sideways Spinal Rocking – Single Knee Hug – Forward and Backward Spinal Rocking – Seated Cross-leg Twist – Child's – Table Top – Cow – Cat – Sexy Kitty – Child's

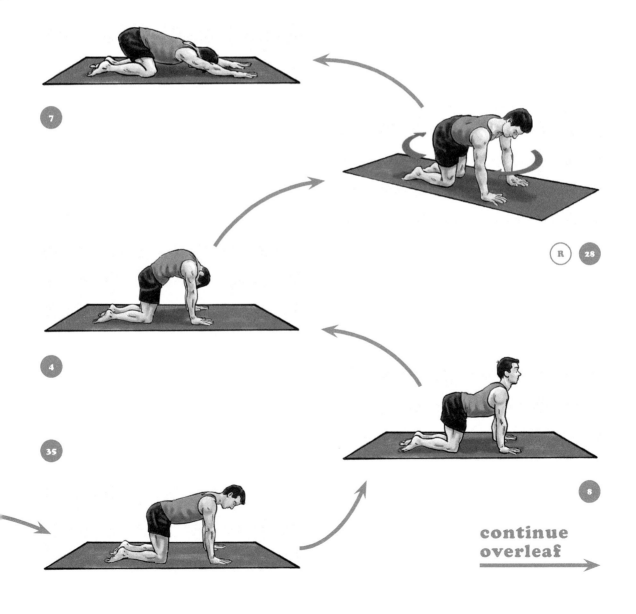

7

R 28

4

35

8

continue overleaf

pink

Mountain – Forward Fold – Half Fold – Plank – Up Dog – Down Dog – Forward Fold – Half Fold – Mountain – Prayer

(For this sequence lead with the right leg, then repeat leading with the left leg before turning the page.)

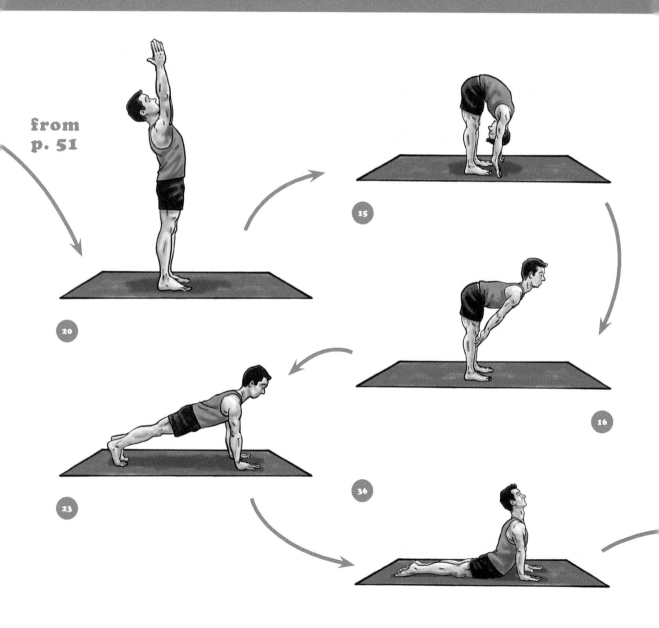

from
p. 51

15

20

16

36

23

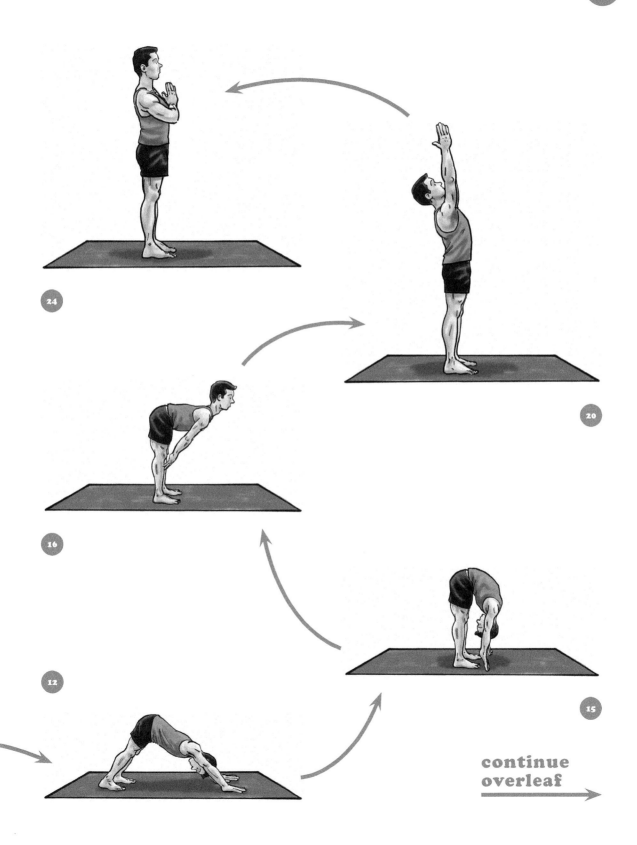

24

20

16

12

15

continue
overleaf

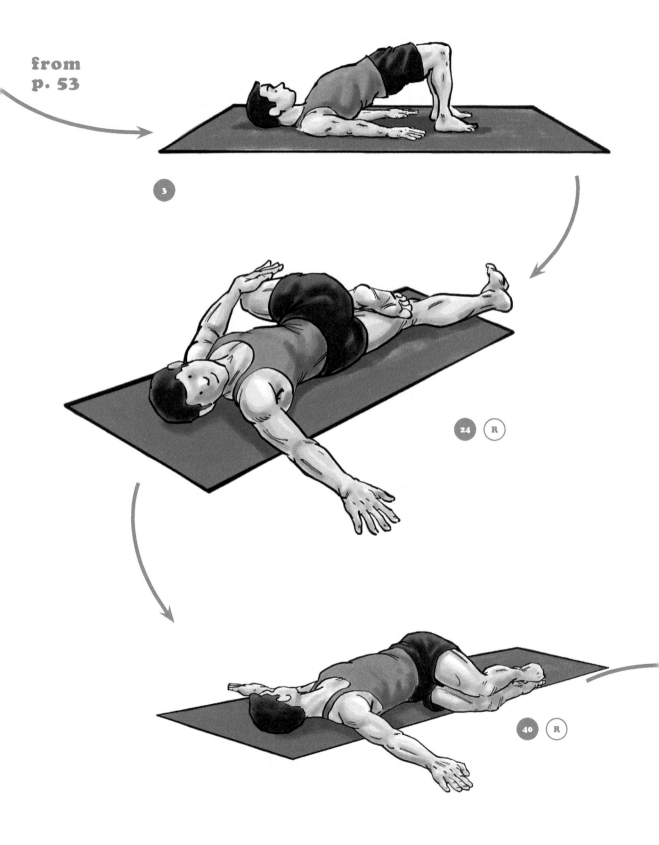

from
p. 53

pink

Bridge – Reclined Single Leg Twist – Windscreen Wiper Twist – Deep Lower Back Release – Corpse

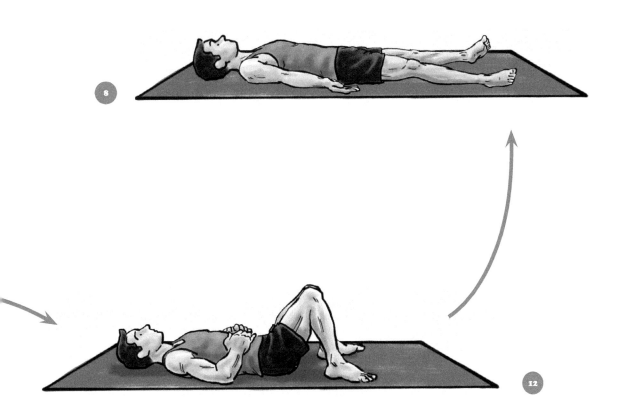

blue

Reclined Stretch – Sideways Spinal Rocking – Single Knee Hug – Forward and Backward Spinal Rocking – Seated Cross-leg Twist – Child's – Table Top – Cow – Cat – Sexy Kitty – Child's

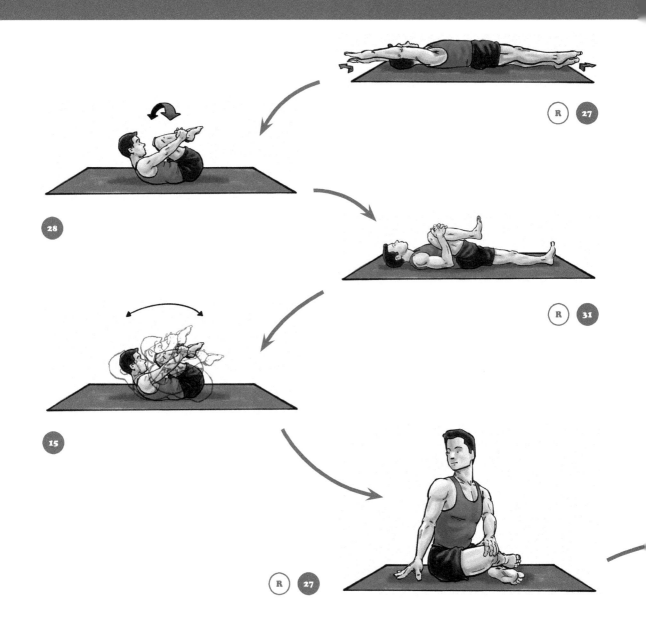

R 27

28

R 31

15

R 27

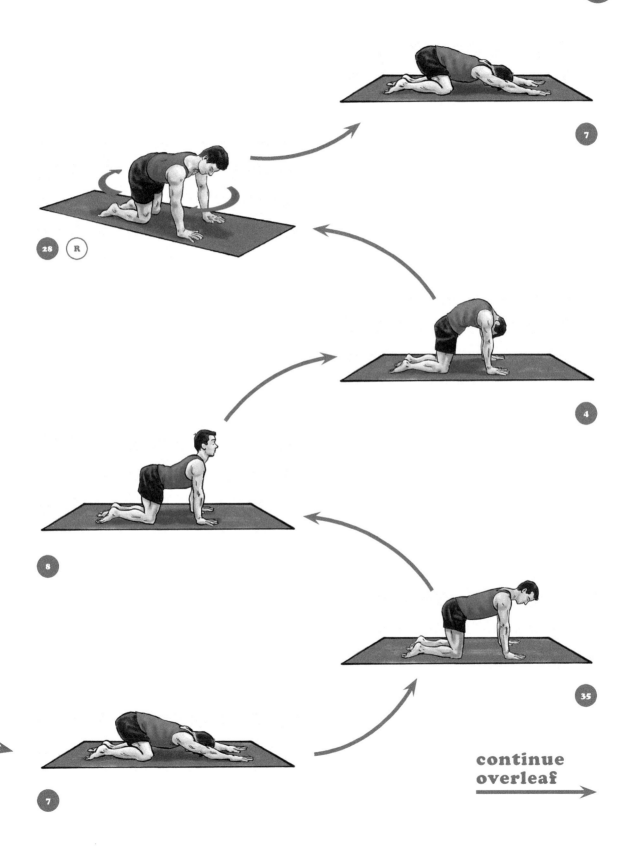

7

28   R

4

8

35

continue
overleaf

7

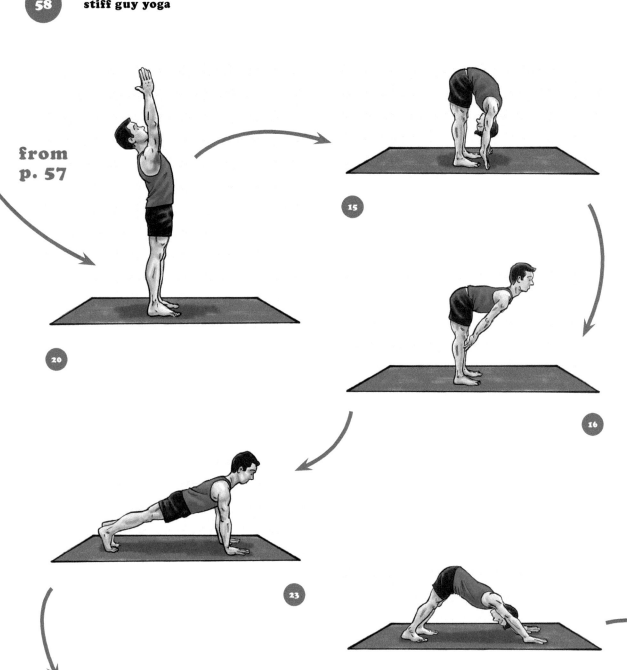

from
p. 57

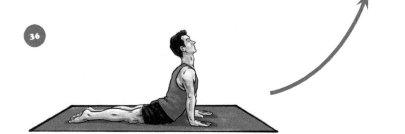

blue

Mountain – Forward Fold – Half Fold – Plank – Up Dog – Down Dog – Forward Fold – Half Fold – Mountain – Prayer

(For this sequence lead with the right leg, then repeat leading with the left leg before turning the page.)

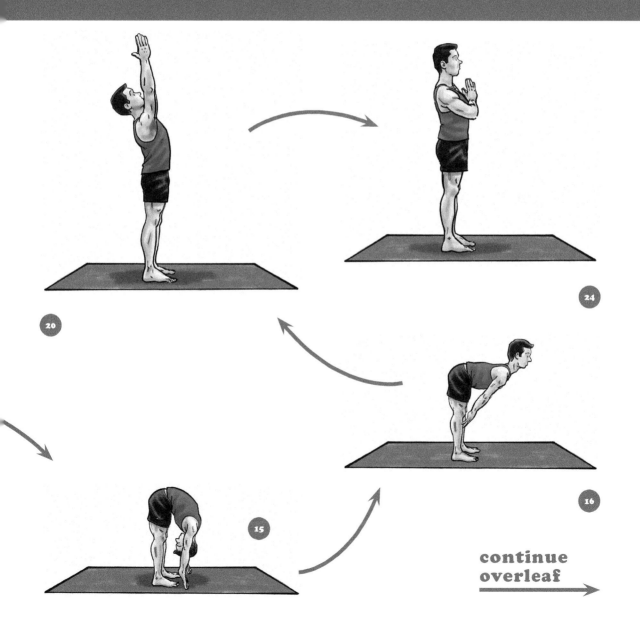

continue
overleaf →

blue

Supported Back Bend – Mountain – Forward Fold – Down Dog – Triangle – Standing Knee Balance – Dancer Prep

(For this sequence lead with the right leg, then repeat leading with the left leg before turning the page.)

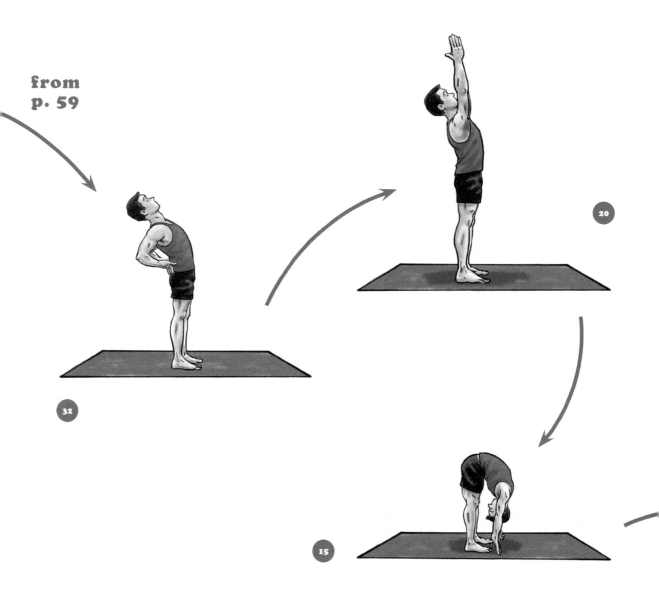

from p. 59

20

32

15

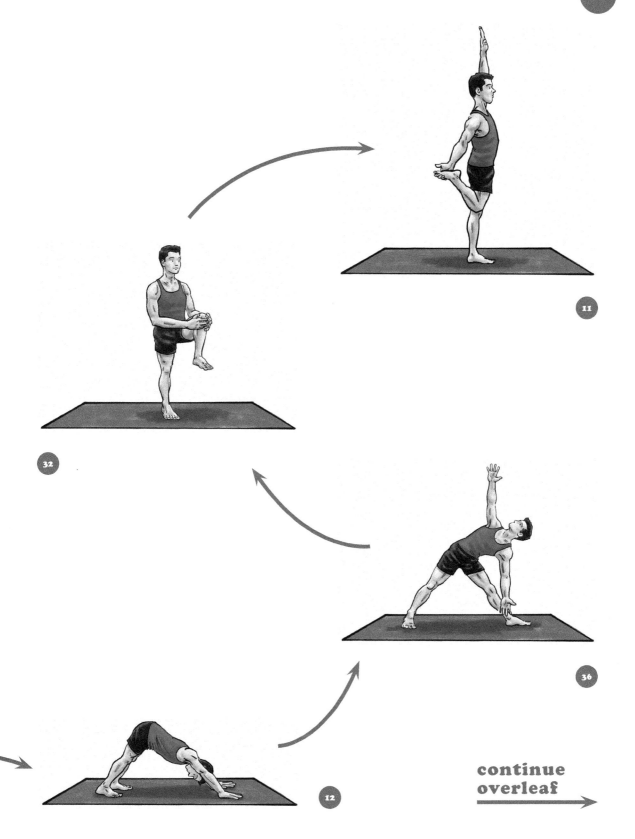

11

32

36

12

continue overleaf

from
p. 61

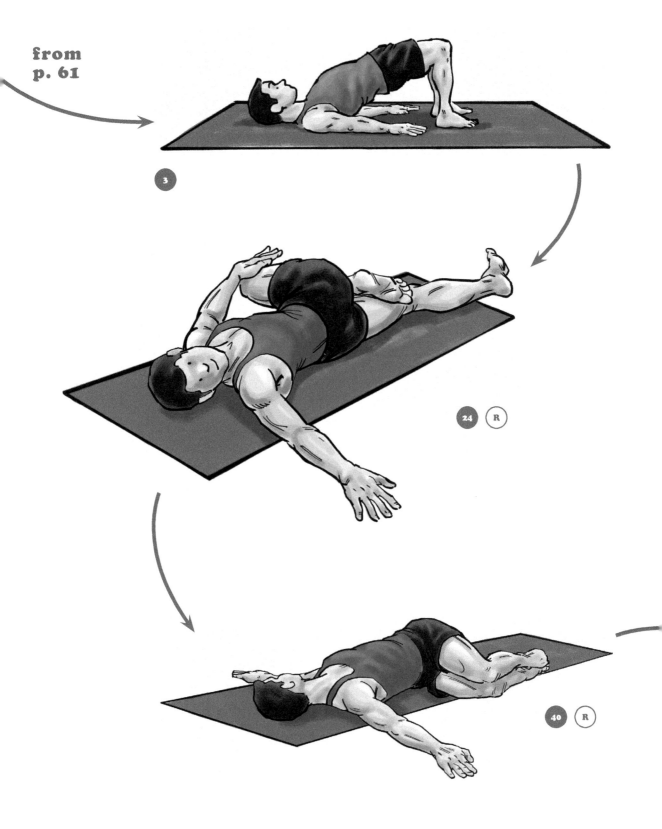

Bridge – Reclined Single Leg Twist – Windscreen Wiper Twist – Deep Lower Back Release – Corpse

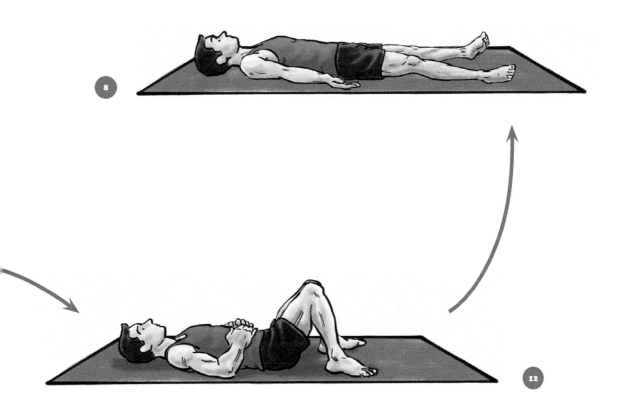

8

12

green

Reclined Stretch – Sideways Spinal Rocking – Single Knee Hug – Forward and Backward Spinal Rocking – Seated Cross-leg Twist – Child's – Table Top – Cow – Cat – Sexy Kitty – Child's

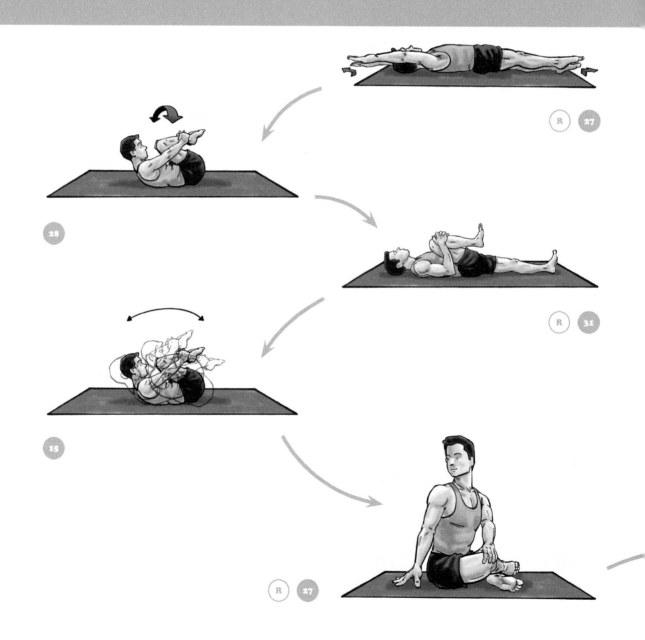

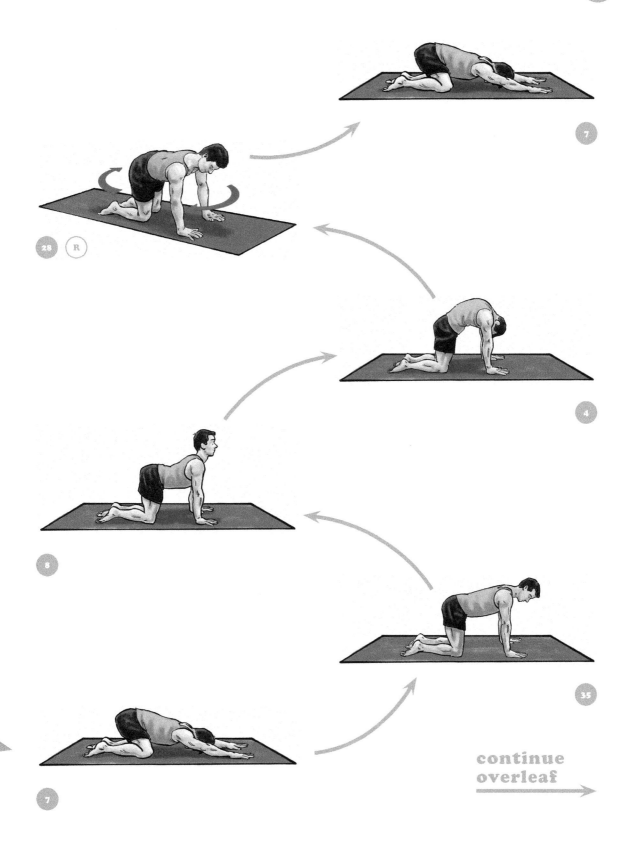

28 R

7

4

6

35

7

continue
overleaf

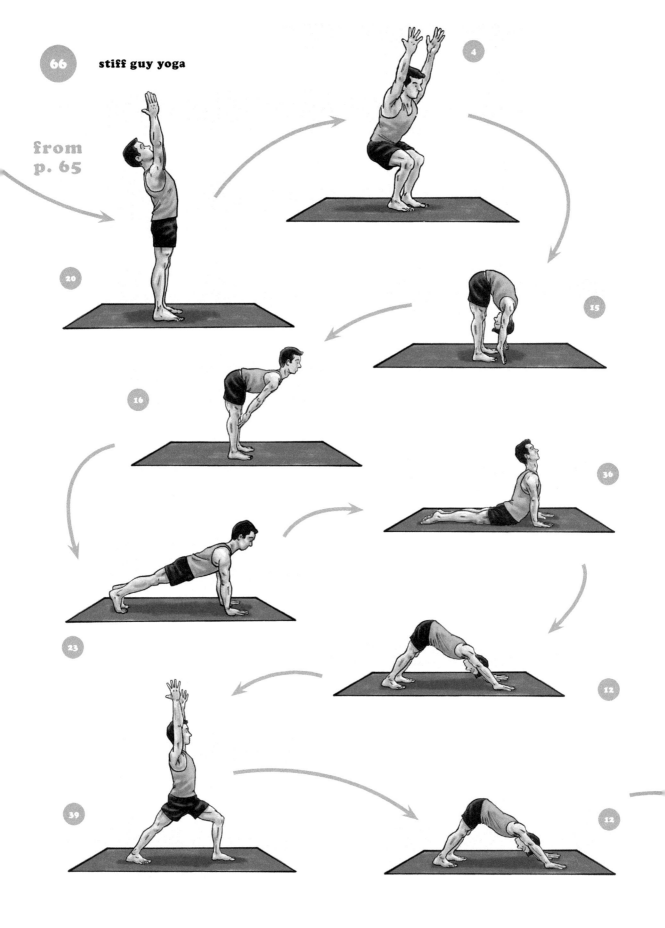

from p. 65

4

20

15

16

36

23

12

39

12

green

Mountain – Chair – Forward Fold – Half Fold – Plank – Up Dog – Down Dog – Warrior I – Down Dog – Pigeon – Down Dog – Forward Fold – Half Fold – Mountain – Prayer

(For this sequence lead with the right leg, then repeat leading with the left leg before turning the page.)

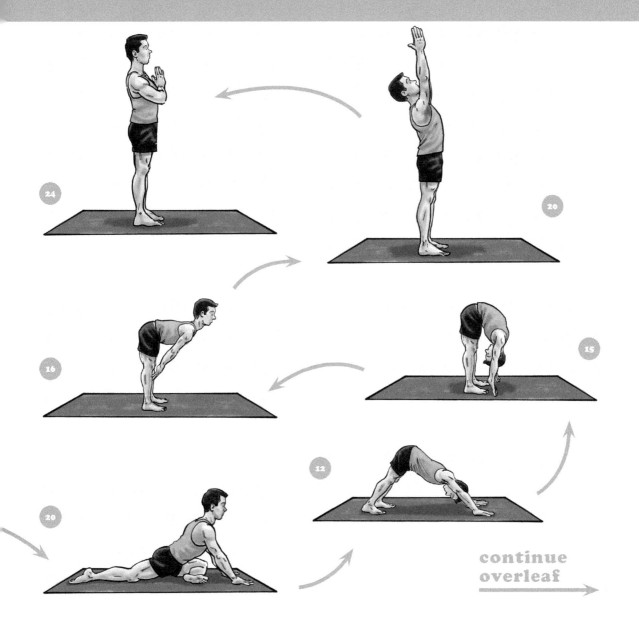

continue
overleaf

green

Supported Backbend – Mountain – Forward Fold – Down Dog – Triangle – Standing Knee Balance – Dancer Prep

(For this sequence lead with the right leg, then repeat leading with the left leg before turning the page.)

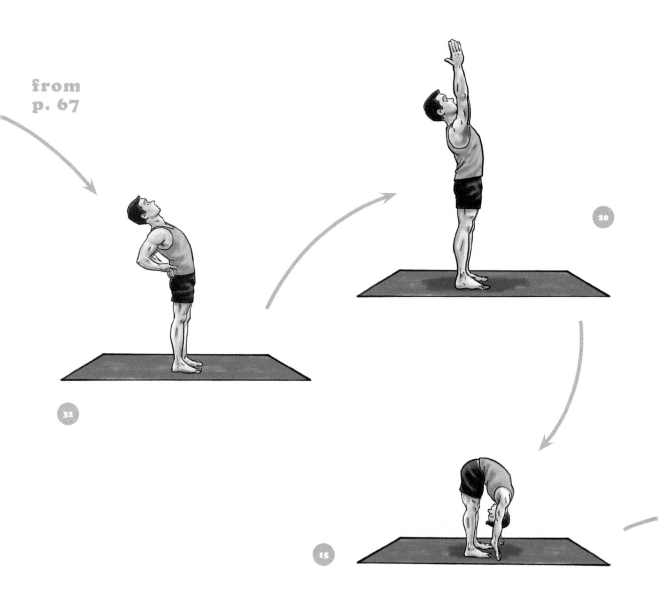

from p. 67

32

20

15

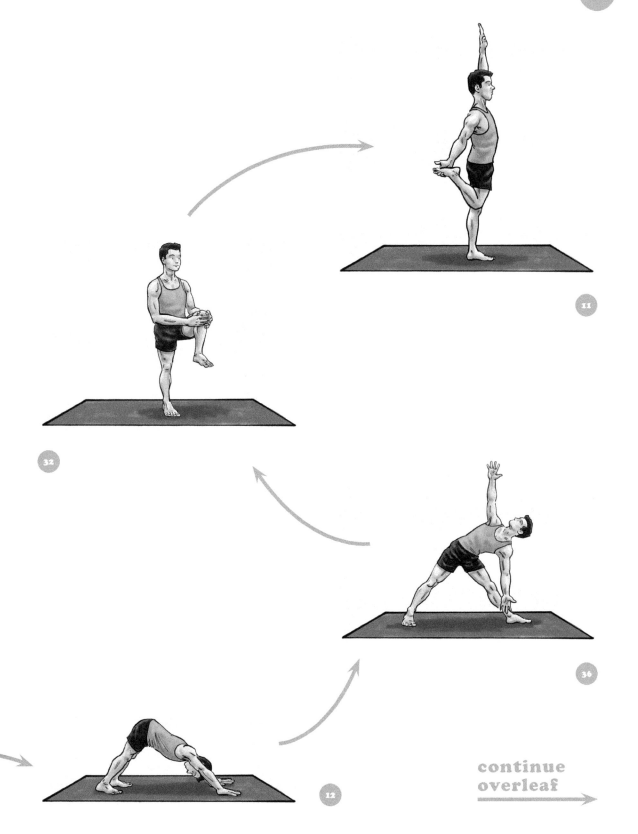

11

32

36

12

continue
overleaf

from p. 69

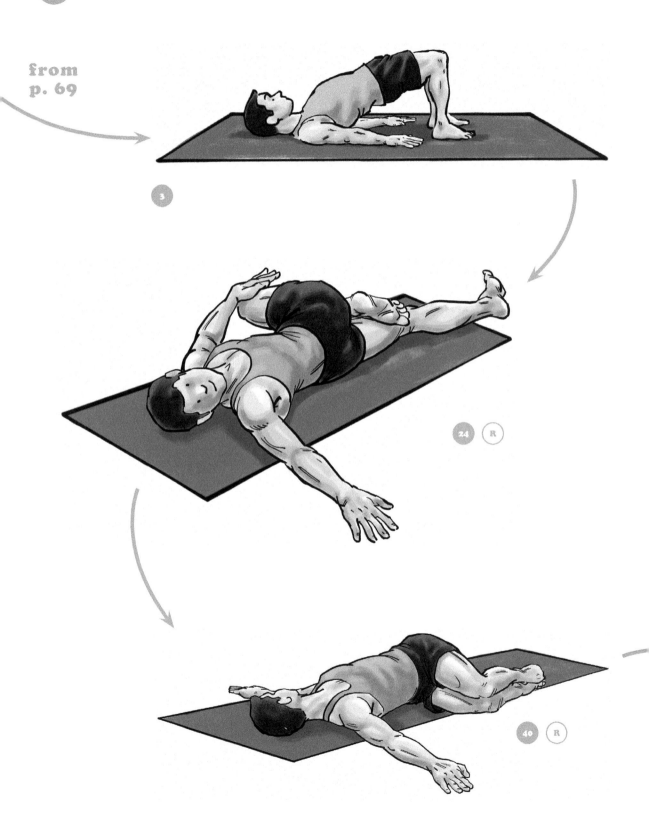

3

24 R

40 R

Bridge – Reclined Single Leg Twist – Windscreen Wiper Twist – Deep Lower Back Release – Corpse

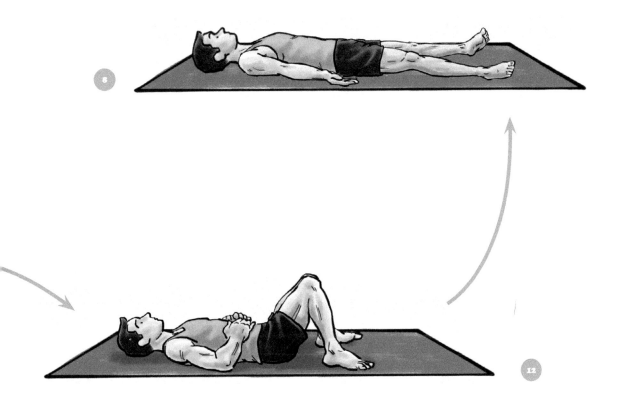

orange

Reclined Stretch – Sideways Spinal Rocking – Single Knee Hug – Forward and Backward Spinal Rocking – Seated Cross-leg Twist – Child's – Table Top – Cow – Cat – Sexy Kitty – Child's

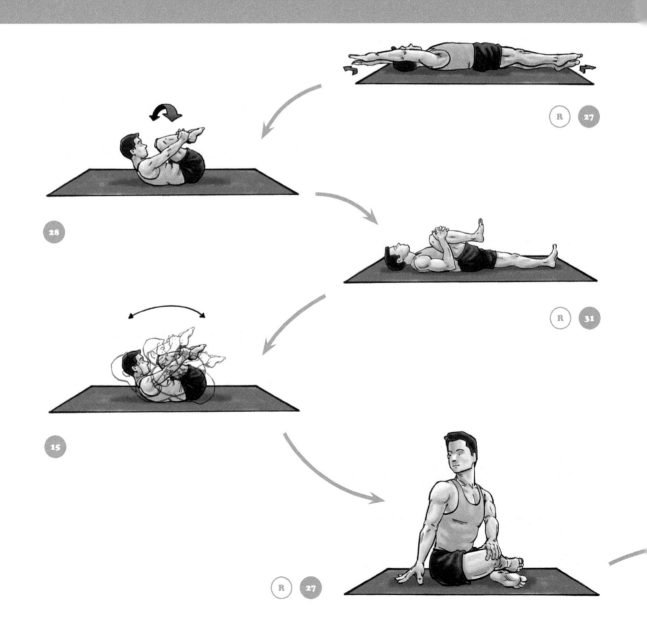

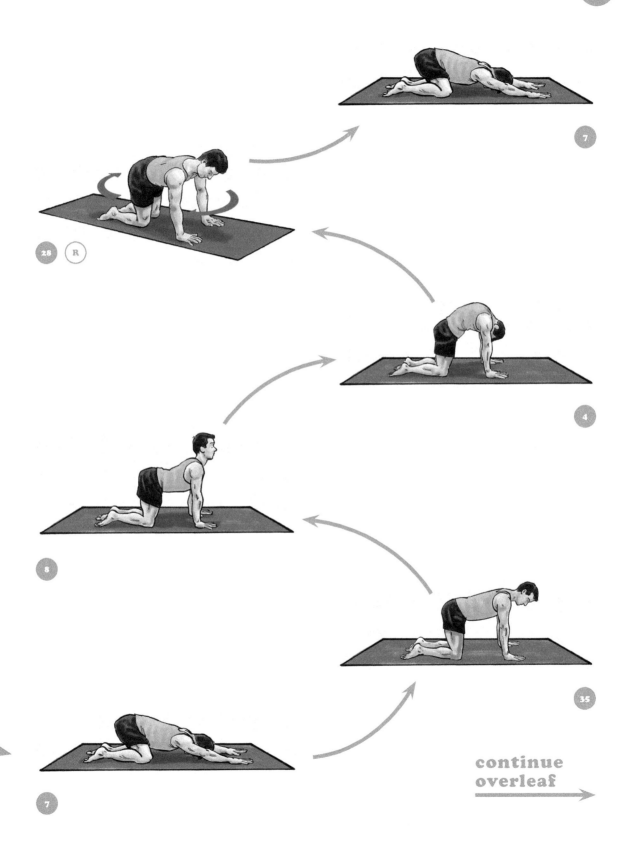

7

28 R

4

8

35

7

continue
overleaf

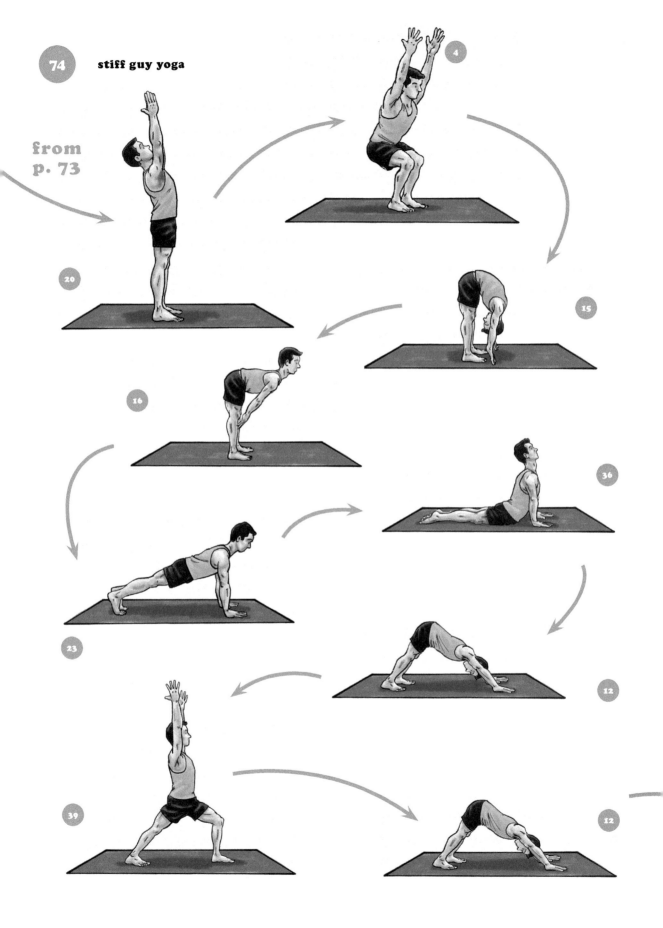

from
p. 73

20

4

15

16

36

23

12

39

12

orange

Mountain – Chair – Forward Fold – Half Fold – Plank – Up Dog – Down Dog – Warrior I – Down Dog – Pigeon – Down Dog – Forward Fold – Half Fold – Mountain – Prayer

(For this sequence lead with the right leg, then repeat leading with the left leg before turning the page.)

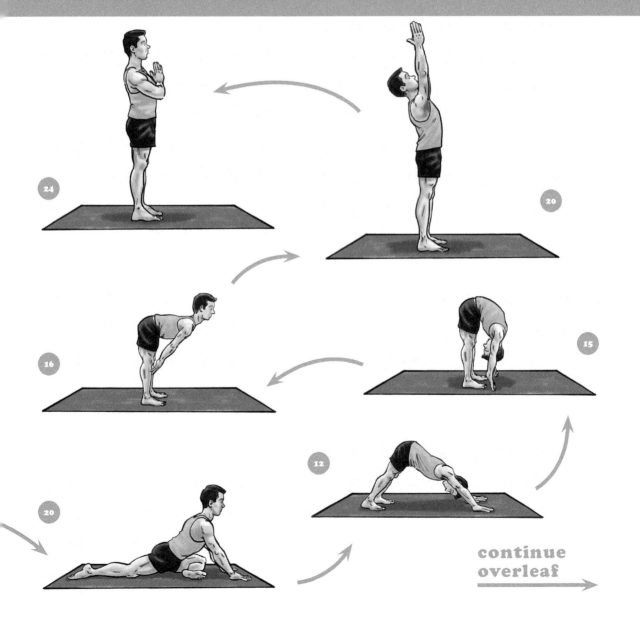

continue
overleaf

orange

Supported Backbend – Mountain – Forward Fold – Down Dog – Triangle –
Tree – Standing Knee Balance – Dancer – Sphinx – Locust

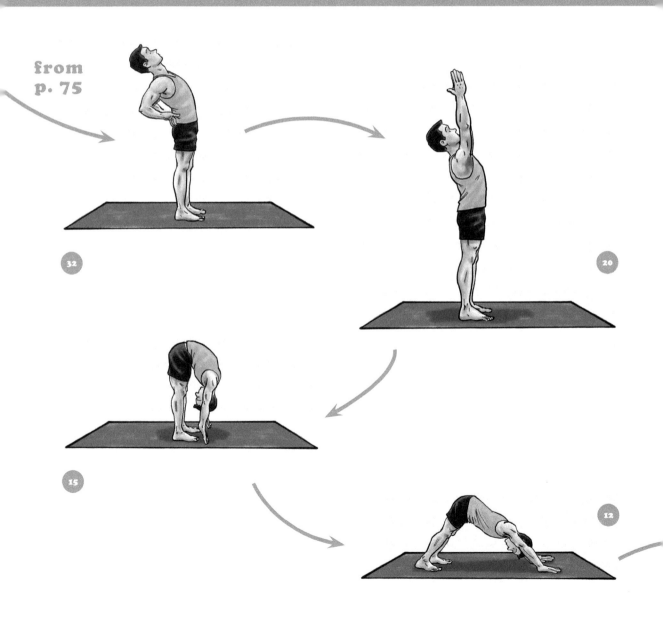

from p. 75

32

20

15

12

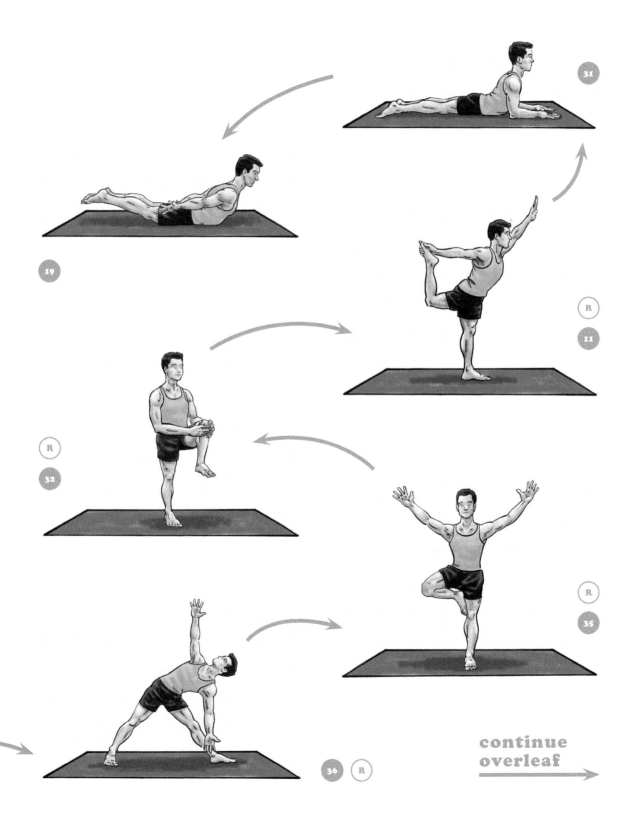

31

19

R
11

R
32

R
35

36 R

continue overleaf

from
p. 77

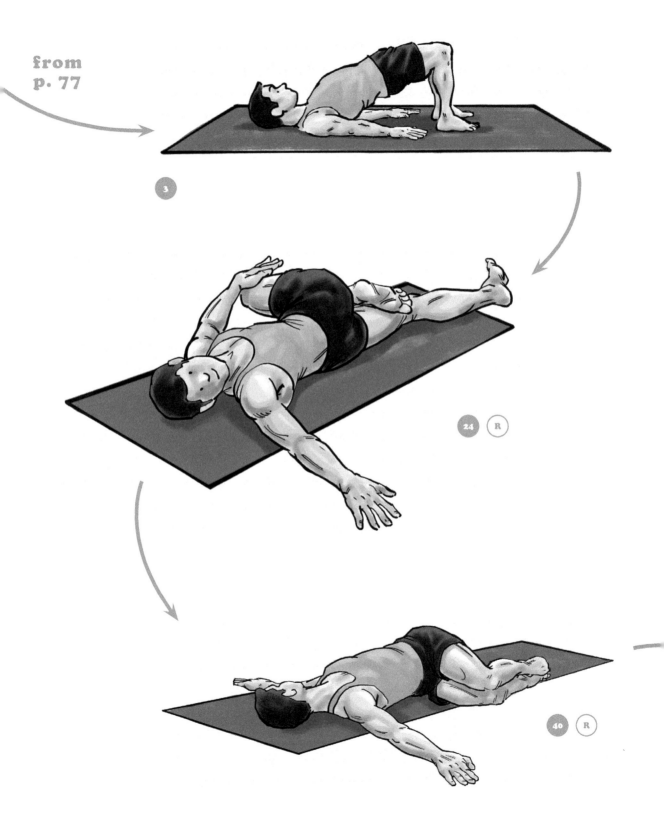

3

24 R

40 R

Bridge – Reclined Single Leg Twist – Windscreen Wiper Twist – Deep Lower Back Release – Corpse

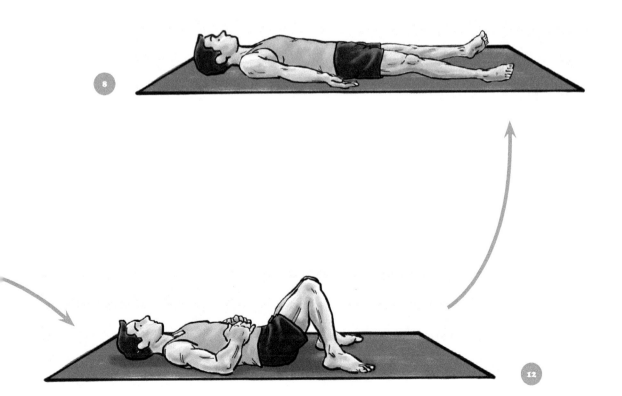

Reclined Stretch – Sideways Spinal Rocking – Single Knee Hug – Forward and Backward Spinal Rocking – Seated Cross-leg Twist – Child's – Table Top – Cow – Cat – Sexy Kitty – Child's

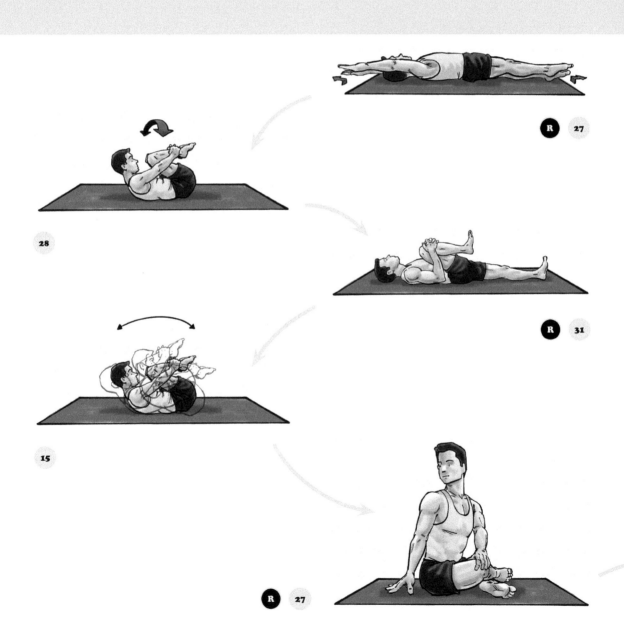

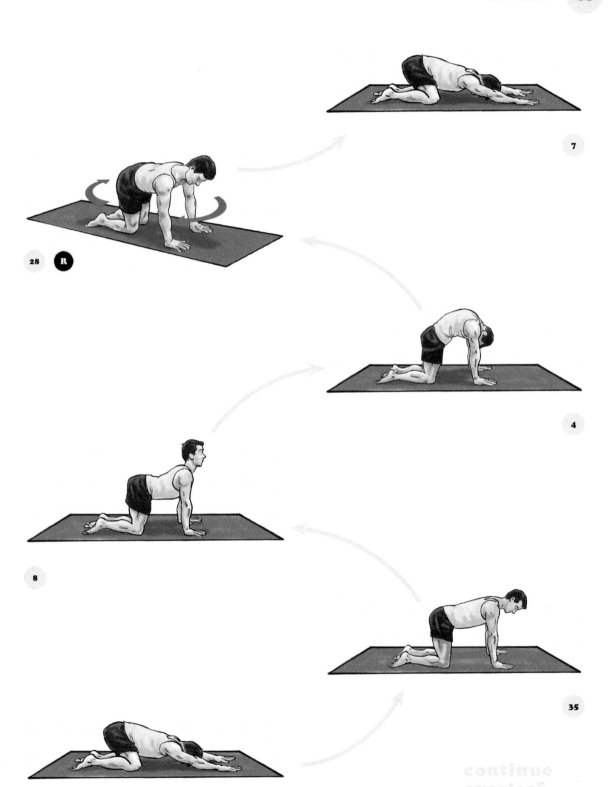

7

28 R

4

8

35

7

continue overleaf

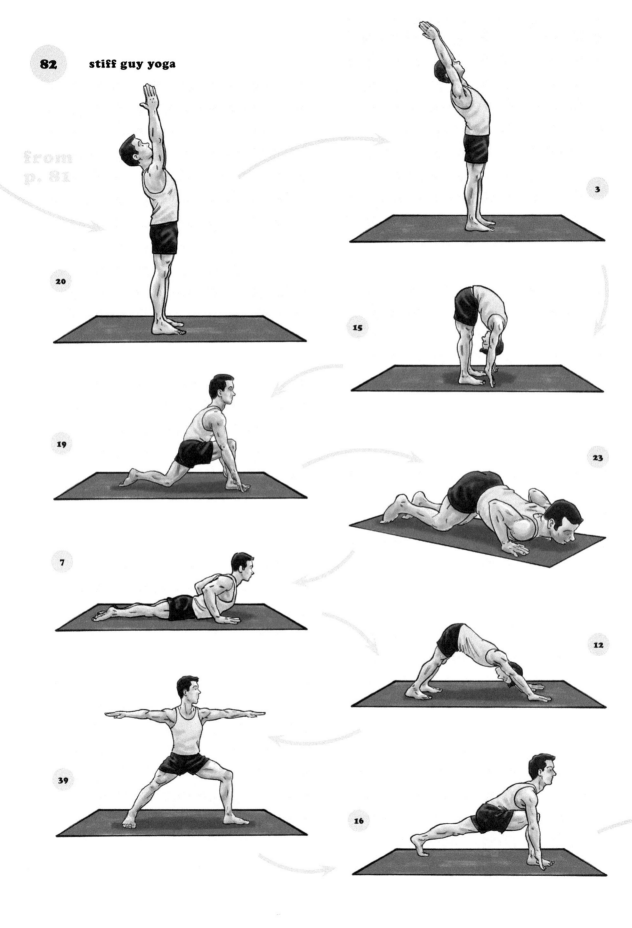

from
p. 81

yellow

Mountain – Backbend – Forward Fold – Low Lunge – Pose of Eight Curves – Cobra – Down Dog – Warrior II – High Lunge – Forward Fold – Mountain – Backbend – Mountain – Prayer

(For this sequence lead with the right leg, then repeat leading with the left leg before turning the page.)

* from Mountain, first move to Backbend, then back to Mountain before finishing with Prayer

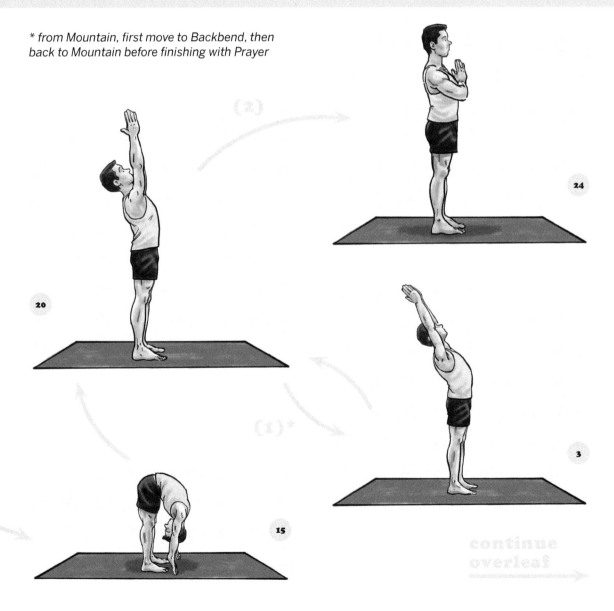

continue overleaf

yellow

Mountain – Chair – Forward Fold – Half Fold – Plank – Up Dog – Down Dog – Warrior I – Down Dog – Pigeon – Down Dog – Forward Fold – Half Fold – Mountain – Prayer

(For this sequence lead with the right leg, then repeat leading with the left leg before turning the page.)

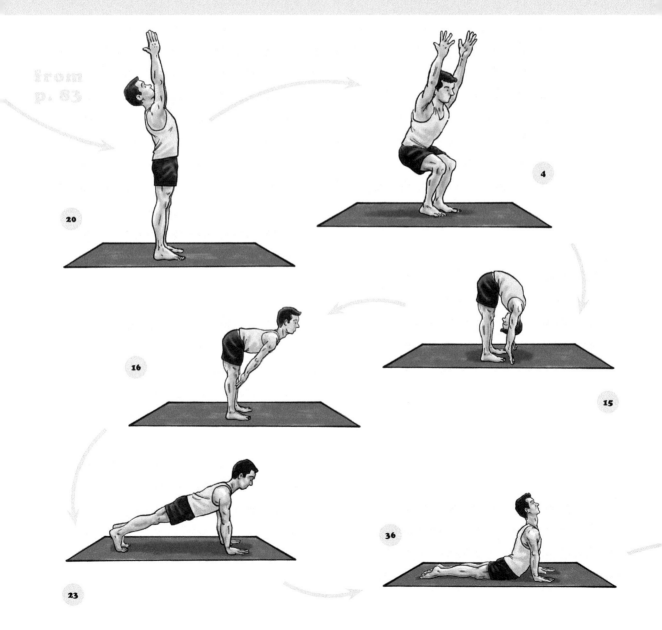

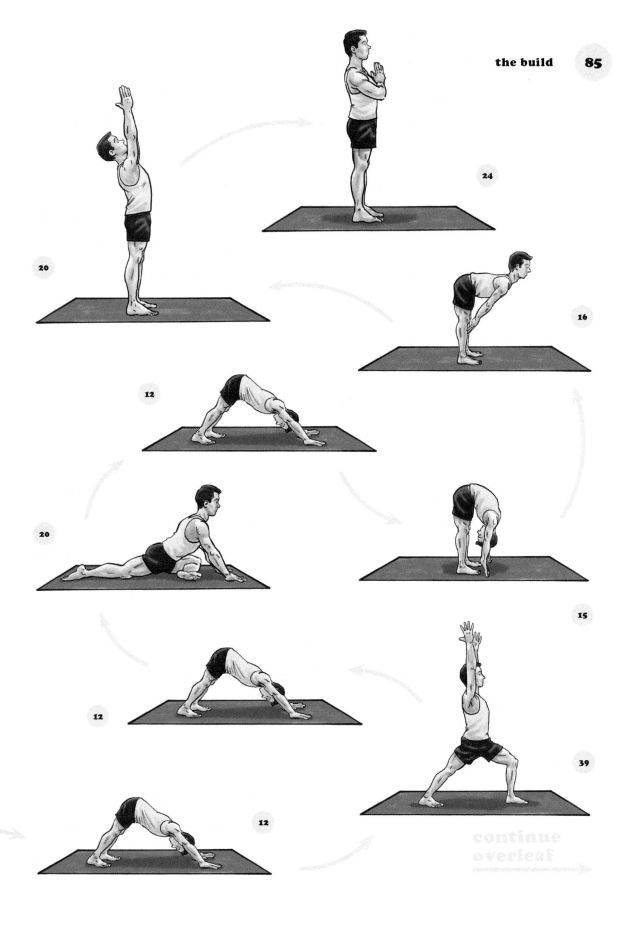

24

20

16

12

20

15

12

39

12

continue
overleaf

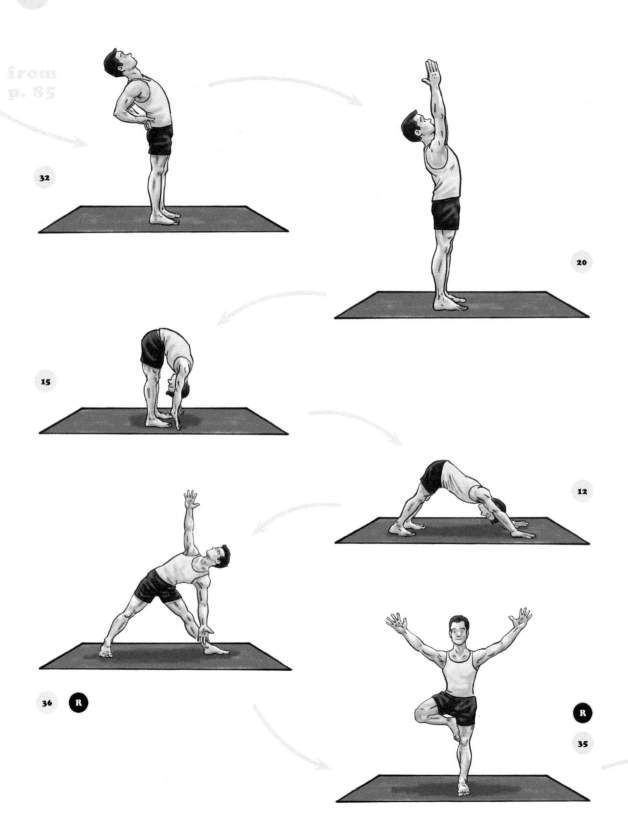

from p. 85

32

20

15

12

36 R

R

35

yellow

*Supported Backbend – Mountain – Forward Fold – Down Dog – Triangle –
Tree – Standing Knee Balance – Dancer – Sphinx – Locust*

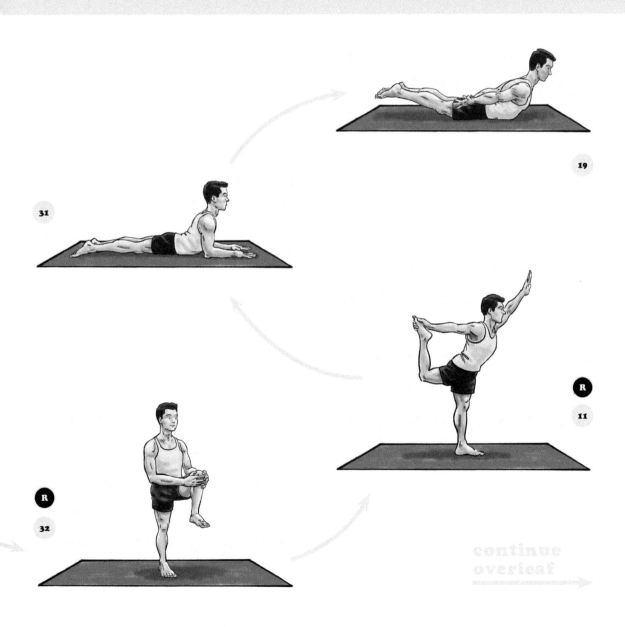

19

31

R
11

R
32

continue
overleaf

yellow

Bridge – Reclined Single Leg Twist – Windscreen Wiper Twist – Deep Lower Back Release – Corpse

from p. 87

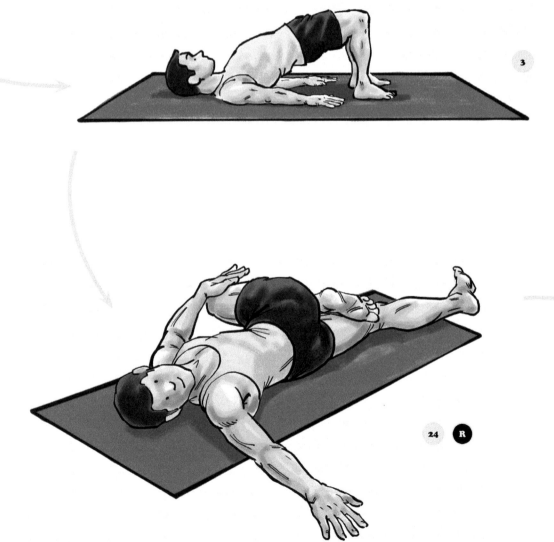

3

24 R

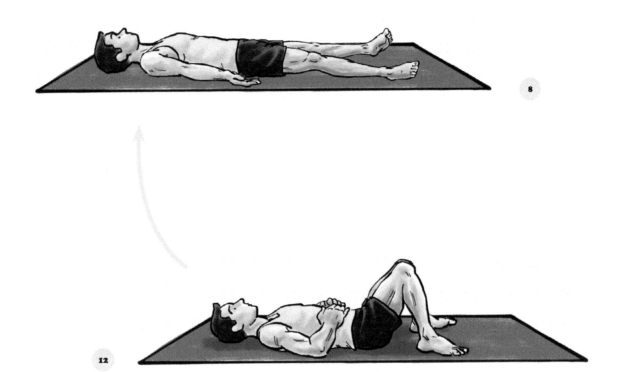

8

12

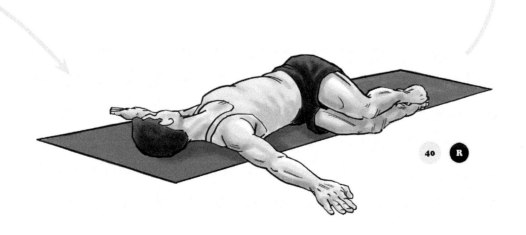

40   R

your twentysomething self

You can weigh yourself until the cows come home or calculate all sorts of numbers like BMI, but the fact is, most of us know what weight we were back when we were young. When we could wear size 30 jeans or a small t-shirt without our guts hanging out. There's a load of great apps out there for tracking weight (a lot of my clients like Happy Scale) and WiFi scales are great for that too if numbers are your thing, but you'll know you're on your way when you find yourself throwing out your clothes and trading them in for slimmer new ones.

Okay, so there's buckets of science about healthy weight. What's really interesting, though, is that the changes I have experienced myself seem to be commonplace amongst others who take up this practise. Let me explain (and I apologise now if this all seems about me, but while the science is interesting, I am interested in real change).

As a lawyer, I worked predominately with men, because at senior level both within my firm and my clients' businesses, there were significantly more men than women at the top. Over the last couple of decades, I noticed a big shift in my colleagues and clients' attitudes towards health. As a young solicitor, client lunches invariably were three courses and always involved alcohol, large slabs of meat and side orders of chips. By the time I'd become a partner, alcohol at lunchtime in the city was no longer the norm, courses were down to one, maybe two, the guys frequently ordered fish and side orders of veg, and gone were the chips. There was clearly a new awareness of both diet and consumption, and guys were openly discussing their weight and health. Something that never would have happened back in the day. And there was no longer the smog of cigarette and cigar smoke which used to pervade not just the dining table but also the office and conference rooms. People don't believe me when I say I can remember the secretaries typing with cigarettes in their mouths! To be clear we're talking the early 1990s, not the 1970s.

Anyway, I digress. Now I'm in the 'wellness' biz, of course diet and health is a daily topic amongst my clients. And I am frequently asked what I eat and don't eat. Well, as I've said, I don't eat meat, but I do eat fish a couple of times a week. I avoid processed food and I cook from scratch. I believe you can have what you want in moderation, so I'm mindful of what I eat but I also try and eat what I need for that day. So, I take account of the amount of activity I've got ahead that day and the times I eat. I avoid, if I can, eating late at night and going to sleep on a full stomach, but obviously you have to fit in with other people. So if I'm meeting friends for dinner, then of course I'm going to be flexible about that. And if I have a day when I've overeaten, then the next day I'll keep things light, to recalibrate.

I drink maybe one or two glasses of alcohol a week because I no longer have the desire for it that I once did. I don't need it to help me relax anymore. And every now and then I'll have a dry month because I think it's good to have a total break. I have also made the conscious decision to reduce my caffeine intake, so the first coffee of the day is regular (maybe two if I need a boost) and after that it's decaf all the way. And you can get really good decaf now, so the taste difference is imperceivable.

I don't have a lot of dairy. I prefer to drink soya or almond milk because I don't like the smell of cow's milk (a hangover of being made to drink milk in the playground, which was blood warm from being left in the sun). And being veggie, soya and nut milks are a good source of protein for me. (But note, unfermented soya is potentially linked to rising oestrogen levels, which isn't great for men.)

Another switch I've made is refined sugar. I used to have a very sweet tooth and now I don't. It took a while and it wasn't easy to start with, but the cravings stopped after a couple of months. So if I need sweetness in something I'm making, I'll use honey, maple syrup or fruit. I also swopped milk chocolate for 85% dark chocolate, which to start with I really didn't like, but with time I became a fan, as it feels a little bit like having an espresso. If you'd like more on getting your food sorted, I have a set of principles and sample meals, plus a list of great resources you can find on my site: www.stiffguyyoga.co.uk.

You don't have to change your lifestyle to do yoga. None of this is a requirement in finding your way back to your twentysomething self, but it's going to change anyway just by practising yoga. The fundamental point is don't stop having fun, but do listen to what your body is telling you and maybe try something new once in a while.

I've made other tweaks and adjustments which I won't go into here, as this isn't about me, it's about you. The reason I mention it at all is so you can see that I'm mindful of what I feed my body. I believe you are predominately what you eat. I know from personal experience that traditional restrictive diets are not the solution. If you need a short-term fix then great, go for it, but long term you need to change your lifestyle. No reason to go mad; just make small incremental changes that you know you can stick to. Start to take notice of what you consume and how it makes you feel. Pound to a penny, you are not really even tasting that lunchtime sandwich that you are cramming down your neck in a rush to get to that meeting.

The good news is you too will change with time. Your yoga practise will give you a greater awareness of your body. You won't need to think about it; it will just happen. It won't be about being judgemental but instead recognising where you are today, and being mindful of your choices, rather than dieting. A friend of mine started Stiff Guy three months ago and has lost over a stone. He loves his beer and I warned him that yoga will affect his intake and he just laughed. He had a work night out and missed his Wednesday class, but was back on the mat for the next class. He was still recovering not just from a lack of sleep, but from the fact that he hadn't even managed to drink half his usual beer quota.

and when you've completed your 30 days

So what do you do after you have completed the 30 days? Well, ideally you should practise yoga two to three times a week, with at least one of those sessions being 60 minutes. Obviously the more you do, the better you will feel, but you should aim to rest your body. Rest is essential for health. It's part of building a strong body.

Other forms of exercise will only add to your health. So you don't need to exclude them. Be smart, use your intelligence and think about what you want to achieve. If you want to run a marathon or do a bike race, then adding running or cycling to your yoga practise is obviously going to help you achieve your goal. Guys are often surprised how much cardio and strength is involved in yoga and how much they sweat. So if you just do yoga you are definitely going to be build muscle, strength and flexibility, but if you want to also lift some weights down at the gym, go for it. Variety is a good thing, as it means your body is constantly learning and adjusting.

I don't do other forms of exercise, but that's because of time and energy constraints. I used to run first thing in the morning, but I wasn't getting enough downtime. I spend a lot of time teaching yoga, and I usually do the class with my students because they find having a visual helpful. So when I'm not teaching, I'm either giving my body a rest or doing my own yoga practise at home, or trying new forms of yoga and techniques in another teacher's class.

This 30 Day Build will be harder than you think. You have to rest. So don't go mad.

bonus material

This book is more than what is written within these covers. You will find more content and supportive material for the 30 Day Build at www.stiffguyyoga.co.uk, where you will find:

- Step-by-step guided video routines for the 30 Day Build
- New video routines for continued practise after the 30 days
- Yoga equipment for sale, including Stiff Guy Yoga mats
- Top tips
- Updates
- And resources that you might find helpful as you progress.

If you want to follow Stiff Guy Yoga's journey, you can do so via our Instagram: @StiffGuyYogaHQ.

And I'd love to hear your stories as you begin your yoga journey, either via Instagram or the website.

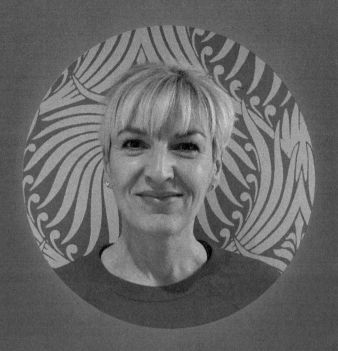

author and illustrator

Nikki Lynds-Xavier was originally a lawyer and partner of a large London law firm, when her love of yoga took her to California to train as a yoga teacher. On her return to the UK, she founded Stiff Guy Yoga, a practice specifically designed for men new to yoga. Focusing on the mechanics of yoga and less on its spiritual side, Nikki's Stiff Guy classes promise no chanting and no requirement to become vegan! Nikki has taught the British Army, the Fire Brigade, businessmen and sportsmen. With waiting lists for her classes and private consultations, and numerous life-changing stories from her students, Nikki was inspired to write this book.

Matt Lawrence's work has been seen on TV, in newspapers and other national publications since the early '90s. When Nikki met Matt, she felt an immediate synergy with him, due to his work as a court artist. Matt has produced illustrations for *Channel 4 News*, *Sky News*, *BBC Panorama* and *The One Show*, covering hearings such as Dr Harold Shipman, Ken Dodd and the Scott Inquiry (Arms-to-Iraq) www.mattart.co.uk.

Little-known fact: court artists are prohibited from sketching in court; it's done from memory, and under the pressure of TV deadlines.